stronger & fitter for life

To my mum, whom I still miss greatly and
who was always there for me.
I hope I've done you proud.

graeme marsh

stronger & fitter for life

feel better ▪ live better ▪ age better

A & C Black ▪ London

First published 2007 by
A&C Black Publishers Ltd
38 Soho Square, London W1D 3HB
www.acblack.com

Copyright © 2007 Graeme Marsh

ISBN 9780713682243

A CIP catalogue record for this book is available from the British Library.

Typeset in MetaPlus by Palimpsest Book Production Limited, Grangemouth, Stirlingshire

Note: It is always the responsibility of the individual to assess his or her own fitness capability before participating in any training activity. Whilst every effort has been made to ensure the content of this book is as technically accurate as possible, neither the author nor the publishers can accept responsibility for any injury or loss sustained as a result of the use of this material.

Text and cover design by James Watson
Cover photos © Getty Images/iStock
Ice skater on p68 and ankle on p70 © Corbis; firefighter on p68 © PA Photos; fall on p71, bend on p80, woman drinking on p116, gardening and dog-walking on p117 © iStock; pelvic floor on p53, clock faces on p74 and p95, golf swing on p80 and blueberries on p124 © Alex Hazle/Axel Design and Photo; all other photos © Grant Pritchard.

This book is produced using paper that is made from wood grown in managed, sustainable forests. It is natural, renewable and recyclable. The logging and manufacturing processes conform to the environmental regulations of the country of origin.

Printed and bound in China

graeme marsh

stronger & fitter **for life**

feel better ▪ live better ▪ age better

A & C Black • London

First published 2007 by
A&C Black Publishers Ltd
38 Soho Square, London W1D 3HB
www.acblack.com

ISBN 9780713682243

A CIP catalogue record for this book is available from the British Library.

Typeset in MetaPlus by Palimpsest Book Production Limited, Grangemouth, Stirlingshire

Note: It is always the responsibility of the individual to assess his or her own fitness capability before participating in any training activity. Whilst every effort has been made to ensure the content of this book is as technically accurate as possible, neither the author nor the publishers can accept responsibility for any injury or loss sustained as a result of the use of this material.

Text and cover design by James Watson
Cover photos © Getty Images/iStock
Ice skater on p68 and ankle on p70 © Corbis; firefighter on p68 © PA Photos; fall on p71, bend on p80, woman drinking on p116, gardening and dog-walking on p117 © iStock; pelvic floor on p53, clock faces on p74 and p95, golf swing on p80 and blueberries on p124 © Alex Hazle/Axel Design and Photo; all other photos © Grant Pritchard.

This book is produced using paper that is made from wood grown in managed, sustainable forests. It is natural, renewable and recyclable. The logging and manufacturing processes conform to the environmental regulations of the country of origin.

Printed and bound in China

CONTENTS

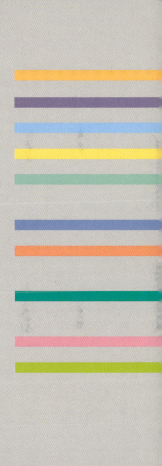

ACKNOWLEDGEMENTS

There are many people who have contributed in some way or another, sometimes unknowingly, to this book. Thank you to you all, but in particular thanks must go to a few people.

To my long-suffering business partner, Greg Smith, God knows how you managed to share a flat with me for two years, and to my father Anthony, an accomplished personal trainer, who is a constant support and counsel to me. Thanks to Lindsay and Su for their help and opinions, to Angela for her astute nutritional input, and my best mate Edward Halls for being such a great friend for all these years.

Thanks to Rob at A & C Black for not putting the phone down on me, Rachel and Amy from the *Daily Express*, whose crash courses in journalism were invaluable, to BBC Suffolk where I first started writing years ago, and to all the editors who I have worked with past and present for your continued faith in me.

An important mention goes to those who contributed to my continued learning, both teachers and students, as well as those I studied alongside. Also, to all my friends and colleagues working in the fitness industry, whose passion and drive helps to inspire so many people.

To all my clients past and present and the awesome team at Aegis Training in London, thank you for the support and constant inspiration you bring me to keep learning and developing. A special thanks to those of you who have stuck with me through changing times and helped make it all possible. You are all a key part of my life and make every day at work a real pleasure. I only hope I have been able to enrich your life as you much as you have mine.

FOREWORD

'Achievement is not the most important thing. Authenticity is. Do not dedicate your life to a concept of what you imagine you should be; rather, be yourself and do not waste energy putting on a performance, maintaining pretence, and manipulating others.

Reveal yourself, instead of projecting images that please, provoke, or entice others. Realise there is a difference between being loving and acting loving, between being stupid and acting stupid, between being knowledgeable and acting knowledgeable.

Do not hide behind a mask, throw off unrealistic self-images of inferiority or superiority. Do not be frightened by autonomy.

Maintain self-confidence, despite losing ground or even failing on occasion. Think for yourself, and listen to others but come to your own conclusions. Respect others, do not be defined, demolished, bound or awed by them.

Do not play helpless, or look to blame, instead take responsibility for your own life. Know your feelings and limitations, and be unafraid of them. Do not be held back by contradictions or ambivalence, and go after what you want. Mostly, have a zest for life, enjoy your work, play, food, sex, and nature, and set yourself up to be a winner.'

Paraphrased from Born to Win, *by James & Jongeward, 1996.*

The above passage epitomises the ethos behind this book. *Stronger & Fitter for Life* is not about looking a certain way or being a certain weight, but it is about being healthy, happy and able to enjoy your life. This book combines years of experience in training and teaching exercise and fitness with a lifelong passion for working with people to achieve their goals. It is balanced with a thoroughly researched base of clinical evidence, proven research and a knowledge of strength and conditioning that spans many genres, from Soviet weight training principles through to Yoga, Feldenkrais, Pilates and many other disciplines.

It is, however, based on the integration of many methods rather than the advocacy of one. After all, there are very few truly 'new' or 'unique' methods, rather there are many different approaches on a common theme. While many health practitioners will champion their method as the most effective, experience tells us that what works for one won't necessarily work for all.

This is the basis of personal training; the task of a personal trainer is to find the right type of exercise for you. By taking influences and techniques from many sources you will have a programme of exercise that is truly personal.

This is what I have attempted to do in this book; although it is not a panacea for all ills, it will allow you to take control of your fitness and find exercises, stretches and routines that work for you.

I hope that the passion and enthusiasm for exercise that went into writing this book comes across and helps to inspire you to achieve health and happiness.

I wish you the very best of luck.
Graeme Marsh MSc MES

HOW TO USE THIS BOOK

The format of this book is very simple: each chapter builds on the previous one, covering a different aspect of fitness, so that you can create your own individual programme of exercise.

As well as forming part of the bigger picture, each chapter contains information in its own right, and you should feel at ease browsing one single chapter if there is a particular subject that is of interest to you.

The book is also designed to be a continuing source of reference for information and direction of exercise, lifestyle, and diet. Keep it handy, so that you can refer back to it for new inspiration, instruction, or direction in your training.

The simplest way to get started is with the self-tests in chapter 2. Take your time to work through each one and record your results. After you have completed these, you will be able to identify some key areas to focus your training on. From there, each chapter will guide you through the reasoning and application of one aspect of the training, beginning with mobility, core stability, balance, movement-based resistance training, cardiovascular work, finishing with nutrition.

Finally, in chapter 10 you can put it all together and design your own programme of exercise. Remember, though, that the book can't do the exercise for you, and it will take effort, application and commitment to get the most from it and reach your goals.

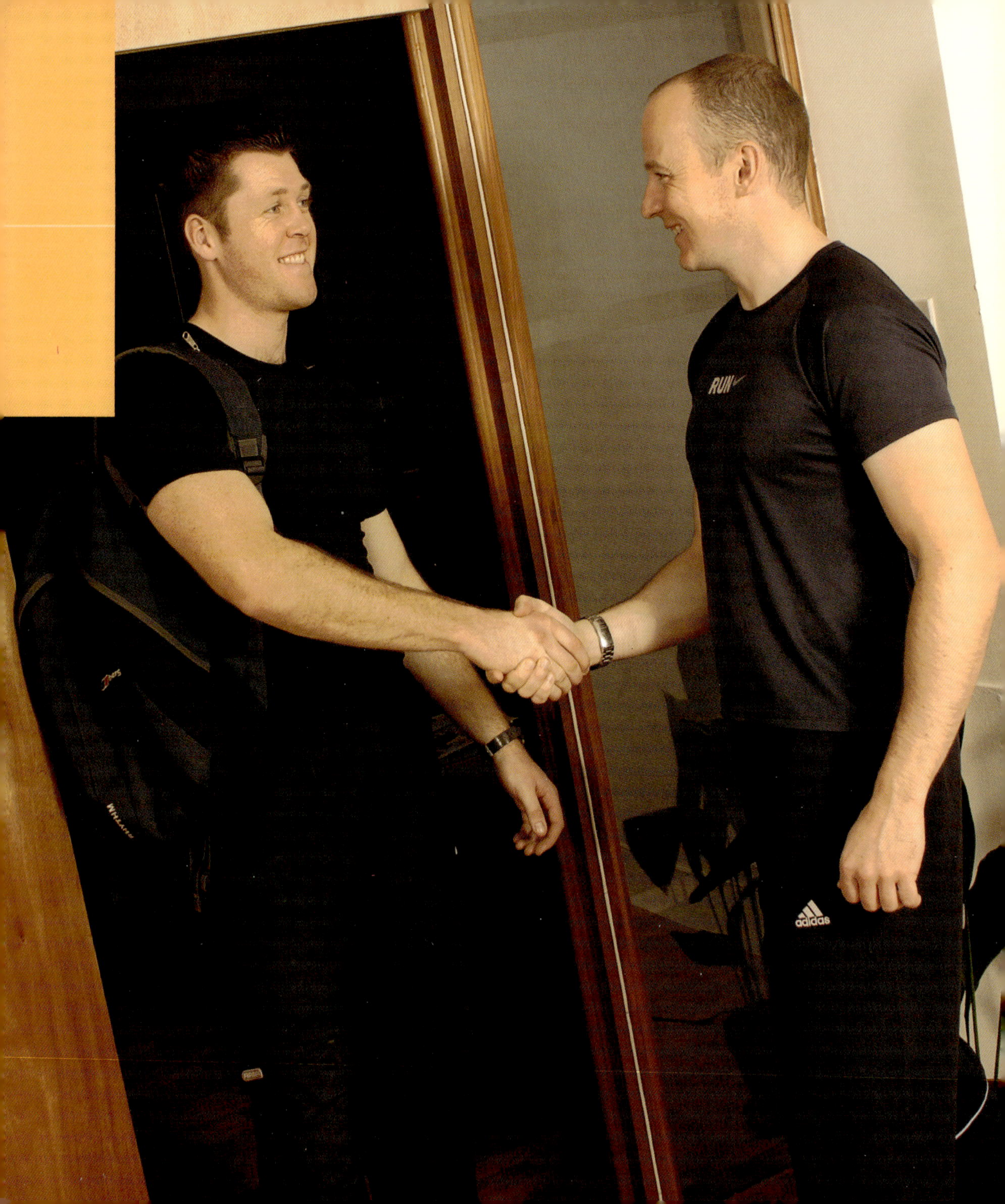
RUN
adidas

Getting Started with Exercise

1

It is no secret that exercise is good for us. Study after study has come back with the same results – if we exercise, we get fitter and healthier, as well as looking and feeling better. We can make a hugely positive impact on our health and lives by using something that doesn't require a prescription, is free of charge to take part in, can be done just about anywhere, and can benefit just about anyone. If you could bottle it, then you'd be rich.

So, why are we getting more and more overweight as a society? Britain has the fastest growing rate of obesity in the developed world. Although we are living longer and mortality rates are improving, more of us suffer from cancer, heart disease and chronic illness than ever before. There are currently estimated to be around a million people with undiagnosed diabetes in the UK, a condition that increases your chances of a stroke by two to three times. Around 40 per cent of men and women have high blood pressure, a major risk factor for heart disease, of which many are undiagnosed. It is a worrying situation and it is not improving.

By taking control of your health, and simply being more active, you can stop yourself from becoming one of the growing number of people living with a reduced quality of life through disease and illness. Not only that, but you can get more from your life and enjoy all the great benefits that come from just getting up and doing something active.

If you're thinking that it all seems a bit daunting and that getting fit means tight lycra, loud music and crowded gyms, then you couldn't be more wrong. By just taking a regular walk, playing some sport or doing tai-chi, you can make a significant difference to your life.

Stronger & Fitter for Life will help you to benefit from having your own personalised exercise programme, tailored to your body through a series of simple self-tests. Unlike many books that focus on weight loss or miracle diet plans, this one focuses on improving function. The exercises in this book are the same as the ones used by some of the country's top personal trainers, and are designed to improve how you move around. I have seen time and time again that, if you improve how someone's body and mind work, their appearance will improve too. Look after function and the form will not be far behind.

For ease of navigation, each section of the book is colour-coded and follows a progression, from testing your own fitness through to designing your own personal exercise programme. There are tips and advice on nutrition, and a comprehensive library of exercises to ensure you never get bored with your exercise routine.

Before we get started on designing your programme, let's first consider exactly how exercise can help you improve your life, and cover a few important points.

THE MANY BENEFITS OF EXERCISE

Just about everyone can benefit from taking regular exercise. By taking a balanced approach to your fitness that addresses all the elements from strength to aerobic capacity, you can effect many positive changes in your life.

A complete review of all of these benefits is a book in itself, so to summarise, here are some of the ways that the training programme in this book can help you.

- Prolonged life – Taking regular exercise will significantly reduce your risk of dying from some of the most common chronic diseases that kill people today, such as heart disease, stroke, diabetes, and some types of cancer. A sedentary person is at *twice* the risk of heart disease as someone active.

- Improved quality of life – Exercise has a positive influence on many aspects of our lives. It can make many daily tasks easier and quicker to perform, as well as increasing our performance at work and at play.

- Better state of mind – The benefits of exercise extend well beyond the physical; how we feel in ourselves can be greatly improved. Research has shown exercise to be an effective tool in treating depression, anxiety and insomnia. It has even been shown to help improve the state of mind during recovery from surgery and cancer treatment.

- Balance and flexibility – Both these qualities are significantly improved through exercise, and therefore reduce the risk of injury through falling or taking part in prolonged physical activity.

- Improved body shape – Exercise can change the composition of the body, reducing body fat and increasing lean muscle. By doing this, we are better able to maintain a healthy figure on a long-term basis, increase self-confidence and self-esteem, and function better.

- Slowing down the ageing process – Many of the negative effects of ageing we go through are often more a side-effect of becoming less active. By including strength training and aerobic exercise in your life, you can maintain and even improve many of the body's systems that would otherwise deteriorate with age. See more on this below.

- Preventing and fighting illness – Exercise can't cure everything, but many people find that exercise can greatly improve how they function and feel, allowing them to live a rewarding and active life. It has been shown to benefit an incredible range of conditions from diabetes, asthma, osteoporosis and high blood pressure, to mental illness, neurological conditions (such as Alzheimer's or Parkinson's Disease), arthritis, multiple sclerosis and many others. Remember, if you suffer from a medical condition such as those listed, or haven't been physically active for some time, you should *always* consult your doctor before starting a programme of exercise.

- Increased sports performance – Behind every top sportsperson there is a top conditioning expert, and even sports like golf and snooker are recognising the many benefits that come with increased levels of fitness. Conditioning programmes are helping to reduce injury and better prepare players to deal with the rigours of their activity at all levels of the game.

AGEING AND EXERCISE

We all know that as we get older it can seem harder to stay in shape, but many older people still manage to enjoy an active and rewarding lifestyle, compete in sports, and carry out day-to-day jobs without a problem.

Many of the functions of the body tend to get poorer with age as muscle mass decreases, strength lessens (particularly after about 70 years of age), and balance and flexibility are reduced; our reactions slow and our ability to work at a given level diminishes. But exercise, particularly strength training, can make a dramatic difference and will address many of those changes that other types of exercise won't.

3

Strength training, by increasing our metabolic rate (the amount of calories we use just to get through a day), means that we use more energy all day, every day. It also helps to activate muscles that don't get used regularly, thus preserving them and keeping them working instead of wasting.

Strength training also helps to improve balance and stability – this is really important, as falling over injures many older people, fracturing weakened bones, and reducing mobility and confidence. By improving the ability of our muscles to generate force and to react to changes in balance, we can prevent many of these injuries.

You're never too old . . .

Strength training can benefit just about anyone, and a landmark piece of research in 1990 proved this to be the case. Over just eight weeks, a group of 10 elderly men over the age of 90 took part in a strength training programme. The results were emphatic, with strength gains averaging 174 per cent and walking speed improving by 48 per cent, an overwhelming endorsement of the benefits of resistance training, even for those up to the age of 96.

WOMEN AND EXERCISE

There is no shortage of myth and misunderstanding about exercise for women. Many head straight for the aerobic equipment in a gym, fearing they may gain excessive muscle or lose their femininity if they use any other equipment. Many women are put off using weights because of images of bodybuilders. These concerns are unfounded; it takes daily training routines at very high intensity, combined with a very-high-calorie diet to reach the size many women fear. In addition, men carry a lot more muscle in their upper body and have far greater levels of testosterone, which is a key muscle-building hormone.

Weights are an essential part of any woman's training plan, and although men might be stronger in absolute terms, muscle is muscle whether it is on a man or a woman; in fact, women generally gain strength faster than men. By including resistance work in a training programme, women can greatly improve their body composition, as well as improve bone density (protecting against osteoporosis), reduce injury risk (women have a far higher incidence of knee injury in sport), and improve their daily performance.

Are men so much stronger after all?

When a comparison of absolute strength is made between men and women, men will almost always come out on top. But, when strength is considered in relation to their fat-free mass or actual muscle size, this difference is virtually non-existent. Women also tend to respond better and faster to strength training than men, meaning that perhaps the difference between men and women is not so great after all.

KIDS AND EXERCISE

Resistance training for children has been a controversial topic for many years, although it is becoming more readily accepted that, if done correctly, it can have many great benefits in helping kids maintain a healthy weight, and improving their endurance and fitness. Contrary to popular belief about bone damage, resistance training can actually help prevent injuries in sport.

Resistance training does not have to mean working with heavy weights or performing excessive amounts of weightlifting. It is generally accepted that the many benefits of training outweigh the risks for kids; if that training is done safely and in a controlled way (many modern gyms now have dedicated areas for children to use with supervision), there is no reason why it should not be of great benefit.

The greatest danger with children is pushing them too hard too soon (or when too young). Programmes should be customised and supervised, with particular emphasis on technique and enjoyment. With child obesity a growing problem, it can only be beneficial to involve children in your exercise plans, whether that is joining you for a walk, swim or cycle ride. For many kids it is a new challenge and a chance for them to enjoy being outdoors. But most of all, it needs to be fun!

Finding the right words to say . . .

It can be difficult to know what to say as a parent or grandparent these days, but here are a few simple rules for encouraging activity in your children:

- be positive and enthusiastic;
- catch them doing something well and give praise sincerely;

- reward effort not outcome;
- focus on skills and technique over weights or times;
- adapt to suit the children and be realistic in your expectations.

EXERCISE FOR WEIGHT LOSS

Apart from enjoying good health, looking good is important, too. One of the reasons many people start to exercise is to lose weight and to change how they look. Our society places great emphasis on looking good and frequently provides unrealistic (and often unhealthy) role models for young people in particular to aspire to.

Exercise plays a fundamental role in healthy, long-term weight loss. Fast-fix routines may bring success in the short-term, but in almost every case they are hard to sustain, not particularly enjoyable, and too restrictive in nutrients to be a permanent solution. How many fit and active people do you know on a diet? Probably not many, though I expect you know someone struggling with their weight who has tried diet after diet without any long-term success. Expending calories through exercise is safer, healthier and more palatable than restrictive and obsessive eating. Exercise can help maintain muscle when losing weight – up to 50 per cent of weight loss through pure dieting can be muscle. As muscle is the only thing in your body that burns fat, you need to be keeping it, not losing it!

So, the bottom line is if you want to lose weight and keep it off, then exercising combined with a healthy eating plan is the most successful solution.

KEEPING IT SAFE

For most people, a programme of moderate exercise is very safe. However, there are some conditions that require special consideration before you begin exercising, and it is always advisable to have a check-up with your doctor before you get started.

To help you find out how safe it is for you to get started, fill in the questionnaire on the following page. If you answer 'yes' to any of the following questions, then visit your doctor for advice before starting the programme in this book. Try to answer each question honestly.

1.	Has your doctor ever told you that you have a heart problem?		Y	N
2.	Do you feel pain in the chest when doing physical activity?		Y	N
3.	In the past month, have you had any chest pain when not doing physical activity?		Y	N
4.	Do you often feel faint or have spells of dizziness?		Y	N
5.	Do you have a bone or joint problem (such as arthritis) that could be made worse by a change in activity?		Y	N
6.	Are you currently being prescribed drugs for blood pressure or a heart condition?		Y	N
7.	Are you over 65 and not accustomed to exercising?		Y	N
8.	Are you diabetic?		Y	N
9.	Are you pregnant?		Y	N
10.	Do you smoke?		Y	N

Remember, answering 'yes' does not mean you are not able to exercise, it simply means that you *must* check with your doctor before getting started (the chances are that they will be pleased to hear of your intention to begin exercising).

Staying safe while exercising is largely just common sense. Take things steadily at first and don't try to do too much too soon. Listen to your body while you are training, and if you start to feel unwell, stop exercising straight away. Take heed of any new aches and pains, and talk to your doctor if you are unsure or if something is troubling you.

KEEPING IT UP – FINDING MOTIVATION

For many people, getting motivated to exercise and to keep exercising is the hardest part. If you are reading this book, you have already moved beyond just thinking about it and are taking action, so well done!

Hopefully some of the information above has given you some powerful reasons to get started and stick with an exercise programme. Your health should be your top priority, as without it everything else becomes difficult – relationships, work, family life, social life, and even your sex life, will suffer from poor health. This alone is a strong motivation to keep at it.

However, despite all the benefits, half the people who start an exercise programme drop out within the first six months. To help you avoid becoming part of this statistic, here are some simple guidelines to keep you on the straight and narrow with your exercise plan. Stick to these and you should have all the motivation you need to be successful in what you want to achieve.

SET SOME REALISTIC GOALS

Goal-setting is used just about everywhere – whether by businesses or by Olympic athletes, it gives us something to work towards and to keep focused on. Whether your goal is to lose weight or to run a marathon, by writing your goals down and having confidence in your ability to achieve them you will greatly increase your chance of success.

There is a common method used when setting goals: your goals can be either short-term (to exercise three times this week), medium-term (to drop a dress size in three months), or long-term (to run a marathon next year).

The simple acronym SMART is widely accepted as a good way to write down what you want to achieve, and this is explained below.

S – Specific

The goals you set need to be fairly specific. Anything too general is hard to measure and to know whether you have achieved or not. Let's consider a couple of examples:

'I just want to be a bit fitter' is very vague and general. How will you know?

'I'd like to be able to walk upstairs without getting out of breath' is more specific and related to an everyday task.

M – Measurable

If you cannot measure a target, then how will you know when you have hit it? As with 'Specific', consider the examples below.

'I'd like to be a bit trimmer' or 'I will be a size 12 instead of a size 14'.

The second goal is easily measured compared with the first and is therefore more likely to be effective. You will also notice the use of the future tense to signal intent in the second phrase.

A – Achievable

This one can be hard for you to know, but it is surprising what people can achieve when motivated and dedicated. Be careful when asking others what they think you can do – you may be disappointed or de-motivated by their responses.

Belief in our own ability is what drives us on – just look at any successful athlete for examples of someone with tremendous self-belief. On the other hand, running a marathon next month if you have never exercised is likely going to ask too much, so try to find a balance. Remember, goals can change as we progress; they aren't set in stone.

R – Relevant and rewarding

As we are talking about exercise here, try to make your goals orientated around the exercise environment and your health. Targets that you set yourself will need to be related so you can establish a good reason to keep your exercise up.

Think about how good it will feel to achieve your goal and how you are going to reward yourself when you get there – maybe with a new outfit or by taking a holiday. The reward gives you something to look forward to once you've achieved your goal.

T – Timescale

Finally, when writing down your goals, set yourself a timescale to achieve them by. Working to a timeframe can help avoid procrastination or avoidance and get you focused on moving towards your goal. Remember, it is your time that you are giving up to achieve this target, so try not to waste it.

When it comes to setting goals it's not what we *can* do that holds us back; it is what we think that we *can't*. Set yourself a challenge that you believe you can achieve. Write it down where you can see it, and follow it through.

GET INTO A ROUTINE

Research has shown there are very strong links between establishing an exercise routine and sticking to that routine. A haphazard approach to your training will prevent you from getting effective results. Schedule your training time into your life, whether on a calendar in the kitchen or with your secretary at work; by making a plan to do it, you are more likely to follow it through. Use self-prompts such as Post-it notes on the fridge or a reminder on your computer desktop, or by leaving your gym kit laid out ready the night before for the morning workout.

There is no ideal time of the day to exercise – some people find that the feel-good factor sets them up for the day if they train in the morning, while others prefer it to wind down from the day when the body is warmer (our temperature peaks between 4 and 6 pm). Research has shown that people who train in the mornings do tend to stick to their training better, but it is not always possible with jobs, family and other commitments. The thing on which all experts agree is that doing something is better than nothing, no matter when you do it.

MAKE YOUR HEALTH A PRIORITY

For too many people, their own health doesn't become a priority until they get ill. Until that point they will often compromise their own health by placing it well down on their list of priorities. Of course, we all know that exercise is good for you, as we all know that excessive drinking and smoking are bad for you. Yet that still isn't enough to get people to make a change.

Healthy living is a lifestyle choice; it doesn't have to mean giving up everything you enjoy, but it does have to mean that you start to value your health. We have already discussed the many compelling cases to do this, but *you* need to make a choice that you want to make a change. Once you do, stick to that commitment. Everyone is busy these days and time is always at a premium, but many very busy people are able to find time to exercise. Keeping active will improve your performance and productivity, so it shouldn't be viewed as time that can't be spared or would be better spent elsewhere.

KEEP IT VARIED AND ENJOYABLE

Exercising should be fun and enjoyable; if it isn't, then it will be a lot harder to maintain the motivation to keep it up. Your leisure time is important, so it should be spent doing something that helps you feel good, relaxed and energised. Once exercise becomes a chore, something needs to change, and fast, before you end up stopping for good.

To keep your training enjoyable, try to find someone else to work out with. A bit of company can make exercise a lot more social and the time pass quickly. However, don't let the social aspect detract from the exercise – your workout buddy is there to encourage and motivate you, not to give you an excuse to rest for an extra five minutes, so try to find someone who is also keen to exercise and has similar goals.

You may have heard the expression, 'no pain, no gain'. This simply isn't true; you should never feel any pain when exercising. Yes, it can involve more effort than sitting on the sofa eating crisps, and you need to push yourself to get the most from it, but push too hard and something has to give, so keep to the guidelines set out through this book for intensity and duration, to stay safe.

The environment can make a big difference to how much you enjoy working out. Whether you exercise at home, outdoors, at a gym or as part of a group, each has its own pros and cons. Sometimes a mixture of all of those can help create variety. Health clubs can be quite intimidating to anyone new to exercise; those with less self-confidence may feel happier in the privacy of their own home. Group exercise can be an excellent way to be active, but it lacks the personal touch that you get working one-on-one with someone. The simple solution is to find what works best for you and occasionally try something new and different to keep it varied.

GET SOME CONTINGENCIES IN PLACE

There is an old adage that 'failing to plan is planning to fail', so it can help to think of some possible things that may come between you and getting active. Once people lapse from their exercise programme, it can be really tough to get started again, particularly after a break through illness, injury or holiday.

Busy work schedules and business lunches can make eating healthily difficult, so eat something healthy before you go and then go light when there. This is an example of planning a contingency to avoid 'falling off the wagon'.

When you sit down to write your exercise programme, think about some of the common things that happen to stop you from exercising (bad weather, smoking, cost, childcare, oversleeping, deadlines for work, social functions, peer pressure) and make some contingencies to help deal with them should they arise.

So, that's the talking over with. You have planned your work and now it's time to work your plan and put it all into action. Start by taking the self-tests in chapter 2 to see how functionally fit you are and then move through each chapter learning about the different aspects of fitness that we will be working on. Most of all, get out there and enjoy it. Fitness and exercise should be a passion, fuelled by the desire to improve yourself and others. Look forward to a better quality of life and health in the times ahead.

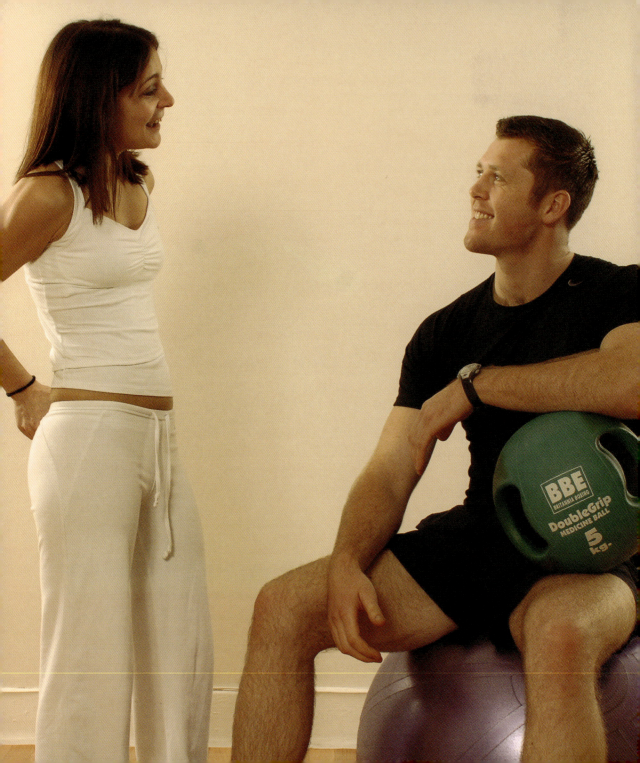

Is Your Fitness Functional?

2

It is a worrying fact that just about anyone can walk into a gym in this country and within a short period of time be lifting weights, running, jumping, in fact just about anything, without doing much more than completing a short questionnaire. Can you imagine going to the doctor's surgery and being handed some pills without first explaining your symptoms or having an examination? Unlikely isn't it? If you are prescribed the wrong drug, the chances are it will have little or no effect, and even worse it could cause you significant health problems. In the same way, the wrong type of exercise for your body won't get you the results you want, and over time could lead to problems of injury and pain. To discover the right type of exercise for you, a few simple tests are needed. These tests can help to identify muscle imbalances, postural concerns, balance and coordination, and areas of relative strength and weakness.

There is a saying when it comes to writing an exercise programme, 'without assessing, you're just guessing'. Although you can't possess the same kind of knowledge and experience as a skilled trainer or physiotherapist, it is still possible to do some simple tests that will help you to select the right stretches and strengthening exercises for your body. By taking these tests, you can identify areas of the body that may hold you back from achieving good movement and, if left unchecked, could lead to injury.

To complete the following tests you'll need the following equipment:

- **a pen and some paper to make some notes;**
- **a piece of string long enough to tie around your waist;**
- **a full length mirror or, even better, someone to take some pictures of you;**
- **a stopwatch.**

Work through the tests from start to finish, as they do progress in a logical order. Remember there is no right or wrong result for each one, as each person will have different answers. Answer each question objectively, based on what you see, and feel free to consult a friend or family member on their opinion as well; two pairs of eyes are better than one! Try to avoid going for what you feel is the 'right' answer, as this will just lead to what is known as a 'false positive' and result in the wrong exercises for you to do.

Once you have completed the tests, fill in the summary box in the appendix on page 142; this will help you to identify the essential exercises for your exercise programme!

TEST 1
BELT LINE

The belt line can provide a quick and simple guide as to the position of the pelvis. This is important when looking at posture as a whole. The position of the pelvis can serve as an excellent indicator of muscle imbalances and likely movement patterns.

For this test you may want a friend or family member to take a photograph of you from the side, or you can stand in front of a full-length mirror and perform the test yourself.

Stand with your feet a comfortable distance apart (normally around hip-width). Let your arms hang by your sides in a relaxed fashion. Look at the position of the belt line. To get an accurate result, this test is best performed wearing a pair of shorts that sit naturally on the pelvis and a top that shows this clearly.

Which one of the following statements best describes what happened during the movement?

A The belt line is higher at the back than the front.

B The belt line seems tipped slightly backwards.

C The belt line looks level.

1

1

Results

Excessive tilting of your pelvis forwards or backwards can lead to muscle imbalances and poor patterns of movement. The hips require excellent mobility if we are to move, exercise and play sports successfully. Any limitations in this movement will lead to the lower back having to compensate, which can lead to problems of back pain and muscle tightness.

If you answered

A This may indicate tightness in the *hip flexor* muscles and weakness in the *abdominals*. You can check this using the Thomas test on pages 29–30. This can be remedied by stretching the hip flexors (pages 46–7) and lower back (page 48) and by strengthening the abdominals and *gluteals* (buttocks).

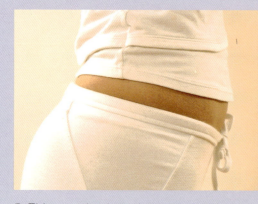

B This can lead to the lower back becoming overly flexible. Over time this can lead to serious problems including

damage to the discs that help protect the spine. Alleviate this by stretching the *hamstrings* and abdominals (pages 47–8) and strengthening the front of the hip using 'Step up and balance' (step-up page 95).

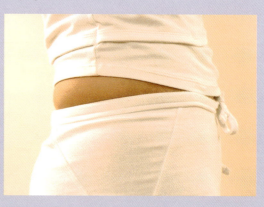

C It sounds like your pelvis is in a good position, which should minimise any stress to the back or hips and help lead to good movement. Recheck this every three months.

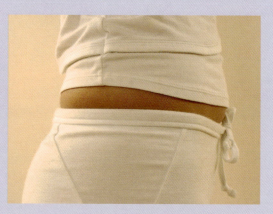

TEST 2
WALL ANGELS

The wall angel is a test for the large muscles of the back and the front of the shoulder. It is important that it is performed correctly to get accurate results. To make things easier, ask a friend or family member to help observe what happens during the exercise. To do this, all you need is a section of wall space around 1m across.

Stand with your heels about 6in from the wall with your buttocks, shoulders and head resting against it.

Place your elbows and wrists against the wall as shown below.

Now try to raise your arms overhead, keeping your wrists and elbows against the wall. As you do this, pay attention to what happens to your lower back.

Which one of the following statements best describes what happened during the movement?

A **I couldn't keep my hands and wrists against the wall without arching my back.**

B **I can raise my arms overhead without arching my back, keeping wrists against the wall.**

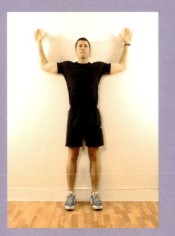

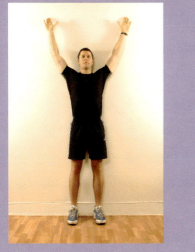

2

17

2

Results

The wall angel is an excellent indicator of the length of the large muscles of the back. These muscles are attached to the upper arm, shoulder blade, and go all the way down to the lower back. Shortness of these muscles can greatly affect stability of the lower back during overhead lifting and needs to be remedied before performing any pressing movement overhead. To help protect your back and to prevent instability, the abdominals also need strengthening.

If you answered

A You are arching your back because the back muscles are tight and short. This can lead to shoulder and back problems when lifting things over your head. Improve the length of these muscles using the lat stretch on page 45 and by strengthening your abdominals.

B Excellent! Your back muscles show good length and this will help prevent injury to your shoulder or back when working lifting things over your head.

TEST 3

FORWARD BENDING

For this test you will need a piece of string long enough to tie around your waist at belly button height. It should be tied tight enough not to slip down when you are standing normally.

Next, find an object around the house you can comfortably pick up from the floor, something like a laundry basket, a pile of books or a small table. In this example we are using a rucksack. Stand in front of the object and bend down to pick it up, paying attention to what happens to the string as you do so.

Which one of the following statements best describes what happened during the movement?

A The string got tighter as I bent over.

B The string got looser as I bent over.

Turn over the page to see what your results mean.

3

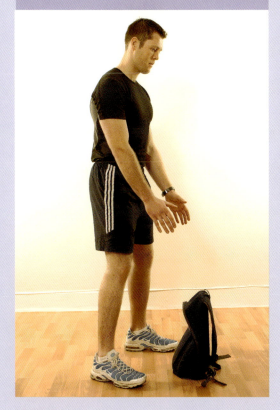

3

Results

The forward bending test helps to see if your abdominals are playing their part in supporting the spine during everyday activities. Repeated movements without the spine being protected can, over time, lead to back pain and muscle imbalance. *Important: if you suffer from osteoporosis, ensure you keep the upper back flat during this movement and focus on bending from the hips. This will reduce the risk of damaging the thoracic spine.*

If you answered

A It's a sign that your abdominals aren't supporting your spine. Begin your core stability training with basic level exercises to master good control before progressing to more complex moves.

B Your abdominals seem to be working well during this movement. By keeping them activated during forward bending, they are keeping the spine well supported. You are ready to take on more advanced core exercises and movements.

TEST 4
SINGLE LEG BALANCE

4

No prizes for guessing the reason for this test. As you can read in chapter 5, balance training forms an important part of your training programme. So, let's get an idea of exactly how good your balance actually is.

Begin the test by standing with your eyes open. Raise one leg off the floor by bending at the knee and hip, ensuring it doesn't touch the supporting leg.

From that position, close your eyes and start your stopwatch. Make a note of how long you can maintain your balance without putting your foot down, hopping, stepping or holding onto something.

Perform this test three times and take an average of your answers (simply add your answers together and divide by three). How long did you manage to balance for?

A **Less than 10 seconds.**

B **Less than 30 seconds.**

C **More than 30 seconds.**

Turn over the page to see what your results mean.

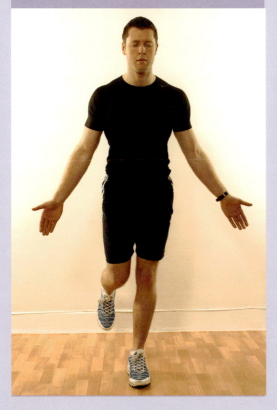

If you answered

A Only being able to balance for such a short time indicates a lack of stability. This means that improving your balance should be a priority in your training programme. Turn to chapter 5 to find out how!

B Though your balance is pretty good, it could still be better and should form part of your training programme. Consider some of the intermediate level exercises in chapter 5 to help improve it further.

C Excellent! Your balance skills are finely tuned and you are clearly very stable during single leg activities. Challenge your balance during the exercises in chapter 6 by performing single leg variations.

4

TEST 5
CERVICAL MOBILITY

Being mobile at the neck is important for everyday activities such as driving, as well as many different sports, including golf and tennis. A lack of mobility in the upper spine can contribute to headaches, muscle strain, poor posture and balance problems.

To check your mobility, first try to look over each shoulder, then try to drop your ear to your shoulder (on the same side). Finally, flex your neck forwards moving your chin towards your chest. Pay attention to how easily you can perform each move and whether you can feel any tightness in the muscles while doing it.

5

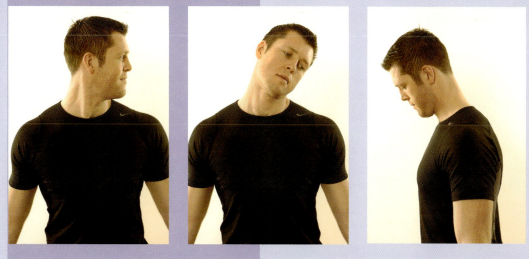

Which of the following answers best describes what you felt?

A All or some of the movements felt difficult to complete.

B All movements felt free and easy to perform.

5

Results

This test can give an excellent idea as to how mobile the muscles of your neck are. Many, in particular the muscles that extend and rotate the neck, can grow tight and restrict movement. When the head position is altered, this can lead to many different problems in balance and function. The neck can also be an area where tension builds which leads to headaches, tightness and pain. Gentle stretching as shown in chapter 3 can help to relieve this at the end of a long day.

If you answered

A Tightness in the neck muscles could be restricting your movements. Gentle stretching can help to relieve this and improve your range of motion. Use the various neck stretches in chapter 3 to stretch the muscles that you feel particular restriction in.

B It sounds like you have good freedom of movement around the cervical spine, but if you suffer from stress or spend a lot of time at a desk you will still benefit from these stretches.

TEST 6
CHEST AND SHOULDERS

The muscles of the chest are particularly prone to becoming short and tight. This is often caused by sitting in poor positions for too long, with the shoulders rounded or hunched over computers. This often leads to problems such as impingement syndrome or frozen shoulder, which can be debilitating and painful. The chest is a classic 'mirror muscle' which people often overwork compared to the muscles they can't see in the mirror.

6

Do this test lying on your back on the floor. Place your hands behind your head without interlocking your fingers, and let your elbows hang down. Ensure you do not arch your lower back as you do this.

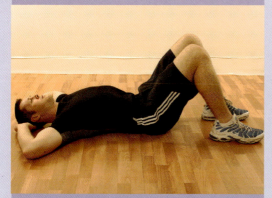
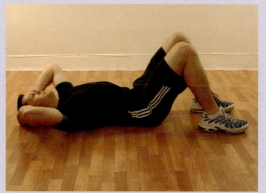

Which of the following best describes what happened?

A **Your elbows and forearms were in contact with the floor.**

B **Your elbows and forearms will not touch the floor.**

Results

Improving mobility at the shoulder is very important to avoid injury. Without adequate movement and balance between all the muscles that control the shoulder, compensations occur that can lead to long-term problems.

If you answered

A Your chest and shoulders are tight and you may have muscle imbalances that could be made worse with training if not remedied. Before your workouts be sure to stretch out your chest and upper back/neck as shown on pages 43 and 44–5. Strengthen using the prone cobra exercise in chapter 3. Also ensure that you perform your *pulling* movements before any *pushing* ones.

B With good flexibility at the shoulder and chest you should be able to easily perform overhead activities without compromising your movements. Recheck every three months to make sure you are maintaining your flexibility.

6

TEST 7
HAMSTRINGS

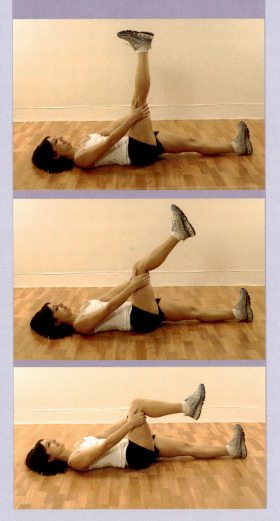

The hamstrings test helps gauge the length of the muscles at the back of the thigh. If the hamstrings are too tight, they can limit movement of the pelvis. This can lead to added compensation in the lower back region, which can lead to injury and back pain. When this happens, the hamstrings can also start to take over the work of other muscles, leading to repeated hamstring strains. See chapter 3 for more information on how hamstring tightness can affect posture.

To perform this test, lie on your back with your hip and knee both flexed to 90 degrees. Keeping the natural curve of your back, slowly try to extend your knee pointing your foot towards the ceiling.

Which one of the following statements best describes what happened during the movement?

A **You are able to straighten your leg fully.**

B **You can almost straighten your leg but not without moving your hips**

C **Your leg stays noticeably bent.**

7

7

Results

Assessing length of your hamstring muscles is important for overall posture. If you found that during the belt line test your pelvis tilted slightly backwards, then it is likely that you have tight hamstrings. This type of posture is explained more in chapter 3. If you find that your belt line tipped forwards then it is not likely that your hamstrings will need stretching.

If you answered

A Your hamstring length is good. Any stretching on this muscle should be done at the end of a session to help maintain good flexibility in this area, but corrective type stretching is not required.

B Your hamstrings are a little tight but probably not enough to cause problems. Ensure that you stretch them after each session and recheck regularly.

C Your hamstrings are too tight! They need thorough stretching before an exercise session to help free movement at the pelvis. Limited pelvic motion will prevent good movements – see chapter 3 for your essential hamstring stretches.

TEST 8
THOMAS TEST

This is a favourite of the physiotherapist and personal trainer for checking the tightness of the muscles at the front of the hip. These muscles have a tendency to become short and tight which can lead to a lack of movement and mobility around the hip and pelvis. You can perform this test either lying on the floor or, for more accuracy, by using a large table. While lying on the floor, bring one knee towards your chest. Take hold of this knee and pull it further towards your chest. Notice what happens to the other leg.

8

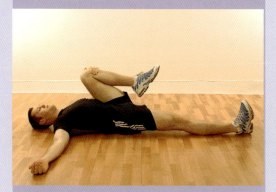 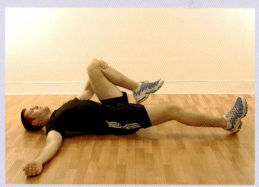

Which one of the following statements best describes what happened to the leg you *were not* holding during the movement?

A Your thigh lifted off the floor noticeably.

B Your thigh stayed in contact with the floor.

Results

Tight hip flexors can lead to problems with many functional activities. This is due to the way that they limit the movement of the pelvis in rotation and extension. This is a common cause of back pain in runners, as running requires a good range of movement into hip extension. Stretching the tight muscles and strengthening the buttocks can often provide considerable relief.

If you answered

A Your hip flexors are tight and they are limiting the amount of movement you have. Before you exercise make sure you stretch them using the multi-plane hip flexor stretch in chapter 3. Tight hip flexors cause muscles of the backside to get weak, so strengthen these with the floor bridge shown on pages 58–9. *Note*: if you suffer from tight hip flexors then it often leads to a rounded upper back, as shown in chapter 3. Avoid doing sit-ups, as this will make the problem worse.

B Your hip flexors look fine. You have good movement at the pelvis without compromising the lower back. Be sure to recheck this every three months for any changes.

TEST 9
CORE COORDINATION

This test helps to identify how your abdominals and core muscles work together with your lower body to protect your spine during movement.

Lie on the floor on your back, with your hips and knees both bent to 90 degrees. Place your fingers underneath the small of your back – you should be able to feel light pressure on your fingers.

Slowly lower one leg towards the floor without touching your heel to the floor. Return it back to the start position and repeat with the other leg.

As you are doing this, notice what happens to the pressure on your fingers.

Which one of the following statements best describes what happened during the movement?

A **The pressure on your fingers lifted, and your back arched.**

B **The pressure on your fingers stayed the same.**

C **This movement caused discomfort in your lower back.**

9

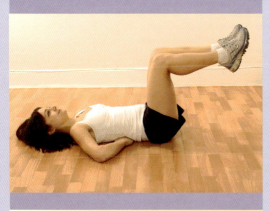

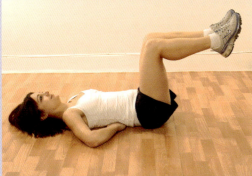

Results

This test reveals if you are able to coordinate the muscles of the core during movements of your lower body. This ability is important during many different everyday activities and also during sports.

Weakness in these muscles can lead to excessive movement around the pelvis, which can lead to injury and back pain.

If you answered

A Your abdominals are not functioning correctly. By improving the coordination of these stabilising muscles with the movement muscles of your lower body, you will feel stronger and more stable during movement. Start with the basic lower abdominal exercise in chapter 3 (pages 47–8).

B Your abdominals are working well to keep the pelvis in a neutral position during this movement. To keep balance in this area, try a version of the lower abdominal exercise on pages 47–8

C If you are feeling some discomfort in your lower back during this movement, it is likely that your core is not func-tioning correctly and there is a muscle imbalance. Start with basic abdominal activation, as shown on pages 57–8. If you continue to feel discomfort see your doctor or a physiotherapist for an assessment.

TEST 10
CARDIOVASCULAR HEALTH

We all know the importance of having a healthy heart and lungs, as explained in chapter 8. They perform the all-important task of getting oxygen and nutrients to our various muscles and organs. They also get rid of the waste products that build up during exercise, such as carbon dioxide and lactic acid. Your heart rate at rest can give an excellent indication of your overall fitness. Many things such as caffeine, temperature and stress can affect your heart, so do this test first thing in the morning on waking.

Locate your pulse – the easiest is the *radial pulse*. To find this, simply turn the hand palm up and place two fingers on the wrist in line with the base of the thumb. Count how many beats you can feel in 15 seconds. Multiply this number by four to get your resting heart rate. For a more accurate result, measure this over five mornings and take an average reading.

What was your resting heart rate?

A **Below 60 beats per minute.**

B **Between 60–80 beats per minute.**

C **Above 80 beats per minute.**

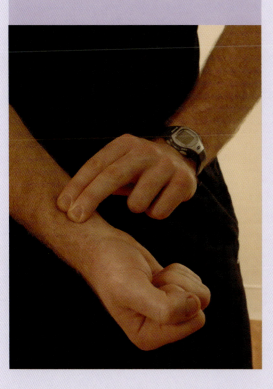

10

10

Results

This simple test of cardiovascular health has been used for a long time. A higher resting heart rate indicates that the heart has to work hard, even at rest, to sustain the requirements of the body. Exercise training can greatly improve the efficiency of this system, reducing the workload on your heart and improving your capacity for exercise. Some athletes have been known to have resting heart rates below 40 beats per minute!

If you answered

A Your heart rate is low, indicating that your heart seems in good health. Make a note of your score for comparison in the future.

B Between 60 and 80 beats per minute is normal for a healthy person. Exercise may still help to reduce this, though, so keep note of your score and recheck it after 12 weeks.

C Above 80 beats per minute means that your heart has to work hard to keep your body functioning. The good news is that through regular exercise you can begin to improve your fitness and ease the workload that your heart is under.

Important note: if your resting heart rate measured over 100 beats per minute then this is known as *tachycardia* and can be dangerous. When the heart beats this fast, it doesn't get time to fill properly, and this can lead to a lack of oxygen around the body (*ischemia*). Before you start exercising, visit your doctor for a check-up.

TEST 11
WAIST/HIP RATIO

For this simple test you will need a tape measure and a calculator. The waist/hip ratio is a simple and commonly-used assessment of the risk to your health from being overweight. This test was recently shown to be three times more reliable than body mass index (BMI) as a predictor of heart disease. Recheck these measurements every six weeks to monitor changes in your body composition and shape.

To calculate your ratio, first measure around your waist at the belly button. Write this number down. Next, measure your hips around your buttocks at the widest point – no cheating! Write this number down.

To get your ratio, divide the first measurement by the second. Check out your results over the page.

11

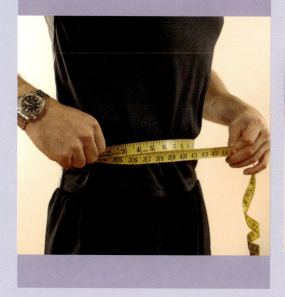
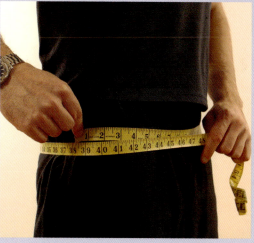

11

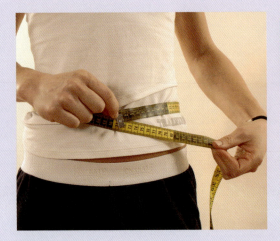

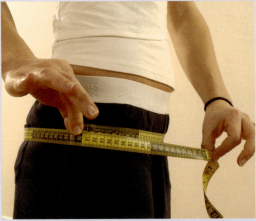

Results

Abdominal fat has been shown to strongly correlate with the risk of heart disease and illnesses such as diabetes. This simple test can be rechecked regularly as your fitness and health improve to show how you are also lowering your risk of ill health in later life.

Men: if you are aged under 60, a ratio greater than 0.9 indicates you are at a high risk of suffering from heart disease in the future. If you are aged over 60, a ratio above 1.0 puts you at greater risk.

Women: due to differences in how we store fat, the numbers for women are slightly different. If you are aged under 60, a ratio over 0.8 puts you at greater risk of heart disease. If you are a woman over 60, a ratio of greater than 0.9 also places you at greater risk.

Even if you fall into the lower risk group, it is a good idea to recheck your waist/hip ratio every three to six months. If you are in the higher risk group, performing the programme in this book will help to improve your fitness and lower your risk of heart disease and illness.

Mobility for Movement – Stretching for Strength

Good flexibility is key to successful movement, and good movement is essential for healthy bones, joints and muscles. As we get older, our flexibility is reduced, and this can lead to a loss of mobility and function, or even injury. As with many other aspects of fitness, this is probably as much due to being less active as it is to getting older. But it's not just age or inactivity that can cause this; repeated patterns of movement such as driving or sitting at a computer can lead to muscles adapting by growing shorter and tighter. As these muscles become shorter, others get longer and weaker, leading to poor posture, restricted movement and often pain or discomfort. The tests in chapter 2 should have given you a good idea of the muscles that you need to work on stretching and strengthening to achieve optimum movement and function.

Many fitness sources advise a generic approach to stretching, suggesting a whole body stretch to 'loosen up' before your session, followed by a general cool-down stretch at the end. This approach can actually make you weaker! Static stretching before exercise can actually reduce the performance of a muscle by effectively switching it off – not what you want if you are trying to really work those muscles. Not only that, but why stretch a muscle that isn't tight before a workout? Surely we want to get our muscles activated and excited ready for exercise? There's more about getting ready for action in chapter 7.

In this book we will look at the reasons why we stretch, and how by taking a more targeted approach to your flexibility work we can get far better results. There is a lot of contradicting information in the fitness industry, and it can be hard to figure out the why, when, and how of

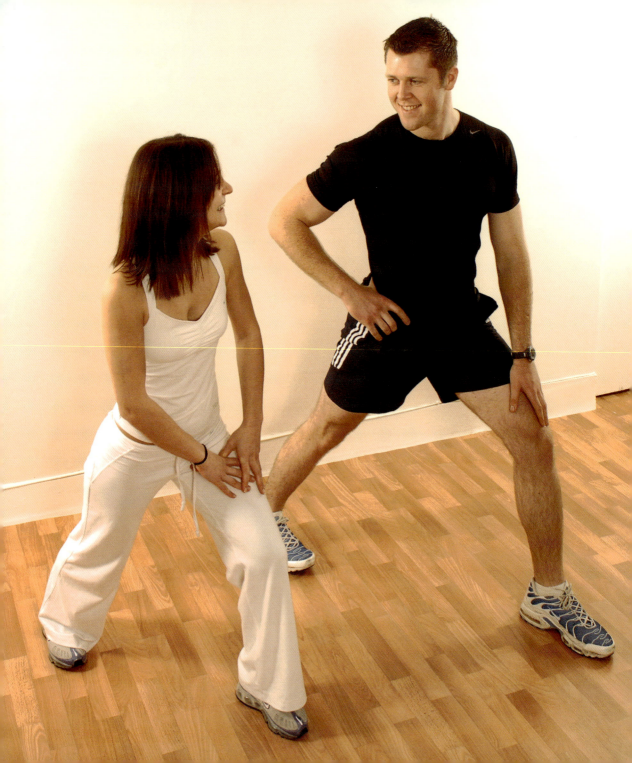

stretching. However, it needn't be complicated; this chapter will help to simplify the science of stretching work and will explain why we need to stretch, how muscle length affects movement and posture, and when and how to stretch.

SO WHAT CAUSES POOR FLEXIBILITY?

There are many different reasons that flexibility can become limited. One of the most common causes is related to posture. A common example of this is when people spend many hours sitting at a computer. Sitting hunched over a computer for long periods can lead to the muscles in the chest becoming short and tight. Over time this can lead to shoulder pain or backache.

Other causes can be related to illness or disease (such as arthritis), immobilisation after an injury, joint replacements, or gaining muscle (known as *hypertrophy*) without also working on flexibility. However, research has shown that weight training actually increases flexibility when done with a balanced approach. Olympic weightlifters, for example, demonstrate tremendous flexibility to perform their exercises.

TIGHT MUSCLES LEAD TO WEAK MUSCLES

Not all the muscles in the human body are created equally; some behave differently from others. Muscles work together to produce movement and rely on a balanced relationship to maintain good movement. Our muscles need to be long enough to allow our joints to move properly, and short enough to maintain stability at the joint. While certain muscles have a tendency to become short and tight, others tend to do the reverse and grow long and weak. This is one of the reasons why a generic stretching approach doesn't work, as each of us has different needs when it comes to stretching.

When a muscle grows tight, a muscle with the opposite job will become lengthened and weak, leading to changes in posture and movement that can cause pain and injury. Over time, the tight muscle starts to shorten physically, losing part of its actual structure as it adapts to being constantly in a poor position. This is why good movement is so important at the start of an exercise programme. Many people develop chronic injuries (such as knee pain or shoulder pain) some time after they start training, which is often related to repeated patterns of poor movement. Sometimes these injuries don't show themselves until an increase in load, such as running further or lifting heavier weights, causes problems. These injuries can be very difficult to shift and become a real problem – prevention is definitely better than cure in this case.

Through performing flexibility exercises, you can restore muscles to their proper length and correct any imbalances.

POSTURE AND MUSCLE BALANCE

Muscle imbalance and flexibility problems are reflected in our posture. 'Posture' really describes how all the various parts of our body are stacked together and can be seen as a more global view of how our muscles are all balanced to keep us upright. The correct posture forms the start and end point for all our movements and should be given careful consideration, especially when beginning a programme of exercise, as postural problems normally lead to movement problems and this can lead to injury. It's not just our muscles that can affect our posture either – ligaments, tendons, bones and joints all have a part to play in keeping our movements efficient and mechanically sound.

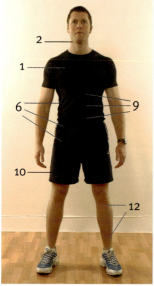 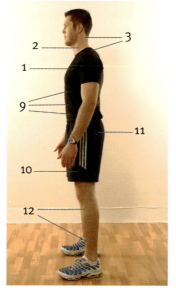 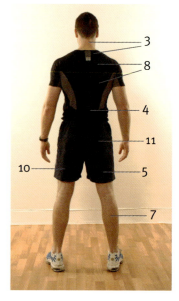

PRONE TO TIGHTEN

1. Pectoralis muscles
2. Levator Scapulae
3. Neck Extensors and Upper Trapezius
4. Lumbar Extensors
5. Hamstrings
6. Hip Flexors
7. Calf muscles

PRONE TO WEAKEN

8. Mid- and Lower Trapezius
9. Abdominal muscles
10. Vastus muscles
11. Gluteal muscles
12. Anterior Tibialis and Peroneals

Poor posture isn't something that happens overnight; it is usually the result of changes that happen over a long period of time. Because of this, it is not always easily corrected, and any exercise programme needs to be supported by changing those habits that led to the development of poor posture. Stretching tight muscles and strengthening weak ones can lead to significant improvements in how we look and feel. Remember that although we should all aim to keep good posture, we are also all different. Some of us are just genetically built better for flexibility than others, so never try to force yourself into a position that causes pain or compromises your posture to achieve a stretch.

HOW TO STRETCH

There are many different methods and approaches to stretching. The simplest to do yourself is known as static stretching. Although there are several other ways to stretch, this method is simple to learn, easy to perform and very effective. It provides us with a good start point and a simple way to stretch the tight muscles in our body that can inhibit good movement. Static stretching works by moving the muscle slowly through its range of movement, avoiding the activation of the reflexes within our body that protect us from injury. To do this, it is important that you always perform the stretches slowly and in a controlled way, avoiding any jerky or bouncy movements; breathe through each stretch to help facilitate a greater relaxing of the muscle.

The difference between stretching and flexibility

Not all flexibility work is static, such as is shown in this chapter. Active flexibility exercises are an excellent way of preparing the body for dynamic activity. In chapter 7, we learn to use active movement as a way of stretching the muscles to prepare them for exercise. These techniques can be used as a warm-up to increase the amount of communication in the nervous system and are far more specific to the exercises we are about to perform. In effect, they are flexibility exercises, as we are taking the muscles through the range of movement that they will be working in during our training session. By doing this progressively, it helps ready the muscles and joints for more dynamic movement.

WHEN TO STRETCH

Static stretching is best used for increasing our range of movement at a particular joint. In this book we are going to use it for muscles that we have found to be tight using our tests in chapter 2.

Since we are using these stretches to release tight muscles, we are going to focus on the use of these techniques at the start of the session, before our dynamic warm-up and resistance training. This way we can release those muscles that can prevent good movement, ready to activate the others. It is best to do this when the body is warm, either after some gentle activity or a hot bath. However, you could also perform these stretches after the workout or at the end of your day for further benefit, as they can aid cooling down and relaxation as well. See more on this in chapter 7.

Warming up before stretching

Conventional wisdom has always advised a warm-up, such as jogging, before stretching. While this is not necessarily harmful, questions remain over whether it is necessary. For example, using *ice* on a muscle prior to stretching has also been shown to be very effective at increasing range of movement at a joint. Much of the research on stretching has heated muscles to temperatures that are unrealistic to attain through a short warm-up and has been carried out somewhat arbitrarily without the use of an assessment to determine what muscles should be stretched in a certain individual. It is also worth remembering that tight/overactive muscles *prevent* ideal movement, and activities such as running require optimal movement in order to prevent compensations and injury.

Getting started

The following stretches all relate to the tests performed in chapter 2. To work at their best they should all be taken to a point of mild discomfort rather than pain. If the muscle feels like it is about to snap or if it is shaking, you have gone too far. This will activate all the body's protective reflexes and prevent the stretch from being effective. Hold each stretch for 30 seconds and repeat each three times for maximum effect. If you are over 65, research suggests that holding the stretches for slightly longer (up to 60 seconds) is more beneficial.

Chest and shoulder stretch

This simple stretch will help lengthen the muscles across the front of your shoulder. This area is commonly tight in anyone with forward shoulders or who has done a lot of pushing movements at work or in the gym. Do this stretch using a doorframe or corner wall.

■ Raise your arm to form a right angle at the elbow with the palm of your hand facing forwards.

■ Place your hand against the doorframe and lightly press your shoulder forwards until you feel the stretch across your chest.

■ Hold for 30 seconds and repeat two to three times on both sides.

■ If you have a stability ball, you can also perform this exercise kneeling (see photo).

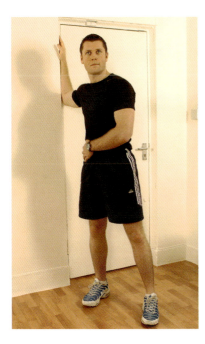
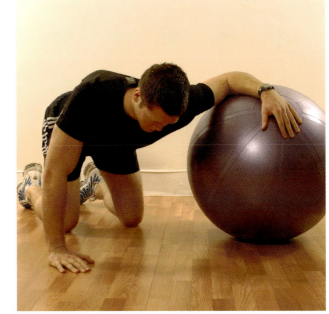

Neck stretches

All the stretches for the neck involve some gentle assistance. Be careful not to force yourself into any stretch. Move *slowly* in and out of each one. These stretches are ideal for anyone with rounded shoulders or forward head posture, which are often caused by too much time spent at a computer or desk.

NECK STRETCH 1 – UPPER BACK/NECK

Sit on a chair or stability ball but do not slump; maintain good posture.

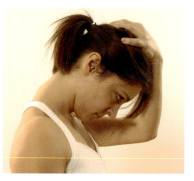

- Slowly allow your head to roll forwards, tucking your chin into your chest.
- *If needed*, to increase the stretch, place one hand on the back of your head and apply gentle forward pressure.
- Hold for 30 seconds and repeat two to three times.

NECK STRETCH 2 – NECK ROTATORS

Sit on a chair or stability ball but do not slump; maintain good posture. Place one hand behind the back of the side of the neck being stretched.

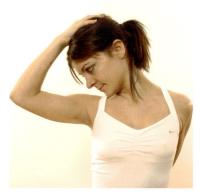

- Keeping your chin tucked in, rotate your head to look directly over your shoulder.
- From that position, drop your chin towards your chest.
- Add gentle assistance by placing your free hand onto the back of your head and move it towards the floor.
- Hold for 30 seconds and repeat two to three times on each side.

NECK STRETCH 3

Sit on a chair or stability ball but do not slump; maintain good posture.

- Lower your ear towards your shoulder until you feel a gentle stretch or resistance.

- From that position, rotate your head upwards, looking towards the ceiling behind you.

- Hold for 30 seconds and repeat two to three times on each side.

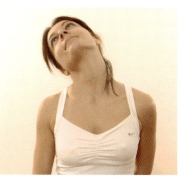

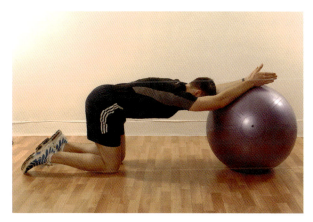

Lat stretch

This large muscle spans the length of the back, starting at the lower back and extending all the way up to its attachment on the upper arm. Tightness in this muscle prevents efficient overhead movement and can also cause an anterior tilt of the pelvis. This muscle has a key function in movements such as throwing, rowing, pulling and chopping. You can use a stability ball for this stretch, or a chair or sofa.

- Begin on all fours.

- With your thumbs turned upwards, extend your arms overhead placing them onto the ball or chair.

- Allow your chest to drop towards the floor, keeping your belly button drawn in.

- Feel the stretch down each side of your body. Hold for 30 seconds and repeat two to three times.

Hip flexors 1

This is a slightly trickier stretch to get the hang of, but done correctly it really hits the spot by stretching the hip flexor muscles through all three planes of movement. There are three distinct parts to the stretch, so take your time moving into each one to get the best results.

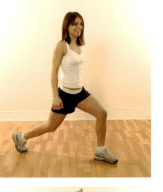

■ Take a large stride forward. Rotate your back foot inwards and keep your trunk upright. Don't let your lower back arch. You should feel the stretch at the front of the hip. Hold this position for 10 seconds.

■ Place the arm on the side you are stretching overhead and slowly lean your trunk away from the side you are stretching. You will feel the stretch increase. Hold for another 10 seconds.

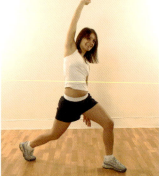

■ Lastly, slowly rotate your trunk and arm backwards. Take care *not* to arch your lower back when you do this. Focus on moving the whole of your pelvis backwards. Hold this position for 10 seconds.

■ Repeat on the other side.

Hip flexors 2

This stretch targets a different hip flexor muscle, and when done correctly you will feel it a lot more in the front of the thigh. This stretch can be done using a stability ball or a chair, or anywhere where you can get your foot to rest comfortably. *This stretch is not suitable if you have pain in front of the knee or kneecap. If so, perform this lying on your side as shown below.*

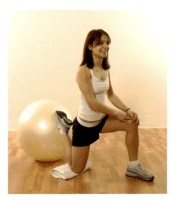

■ Start in a kneeling position with one foot forwards and one back as shown below.

- Place your rear foot on a low chair or stability ball.
- Bring your trunk into an upright position to feel the stretch down the front of your thigh.
- Balance may be tricky at first, so use another chair or stick for support, if needed.
- Hold for 30 seconds and repeat two to three times on each side.

Hamstrings

This simple stretch is the same as the test used for the hamstring muscles in chapter 2. It targets the large muscles at the back of the thigh; these are worked very hard during activities such as running, for which this is an excellent cool-down stretch. Done before exercise, it can help increase forward movement of the pelvis, protecting the lower back.

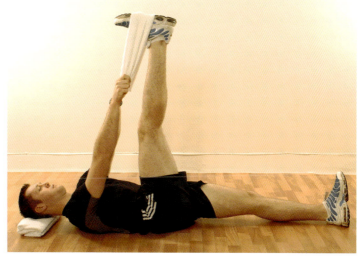

- Start by lying on the floor on your back with your hip and knee flexed to 90 degrees.
- Slowly extend your knee towards the ceiling. Be sure to keep your spine in a neutral position by not allowing your pelvis to tip backwards.
- Hold for 30 seconds, repeat on each side two to three times.
- For an increased stretch, you can use a towel or rope around your foot to help you gently pull your foot towards the ceiling.

Abdominals

It is common in people with a flat back for their abdominal muscles to become short and tight. This tends to depress the chest and lead to rounded shoulders, too. This movement is a mixture of a postural strength exercise and a stretch that combines breathing to improve posture and muscle length by stretching the abdominals and the muscles around the ribcage.

- Stand against a wall with your heels around 6in away from the bottom. Place your arms against the wall as for the wall angel test in chapter 2.

- Slowly extend your arms up the wall, holding at the top of the movement.

- Ensure that your lower back is not arched.

- Take five deep breaths in that position. Begin by filling the tummy first, then feeling your lungs expanding like two balloons.

- Return to the start position and repeat two to three times.

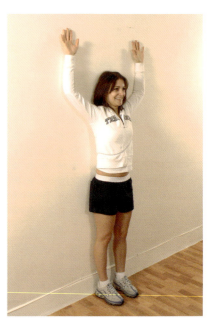

Lower back

If you suffer from lower back pain, injury or damage to the spinal discs, or have had a hip replacement, do not perform this stretch.

This stretch can be an excellent way to relieve tightness in the muscles that extend the trunk. However, care must be taken as it places the back in a position of extreme flexion. It is an ideal stretch for anyone whose pelvis is tilted forward, as indicated in chapter 2.

- Start by lying on the floor, slowly drawing your knees up towards your chest.

- Slowly rock backwards, bringing your backside up from the floor.

- Hold for 30 seconds and repeat two to three times.

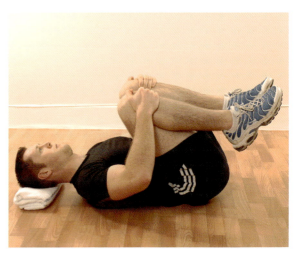

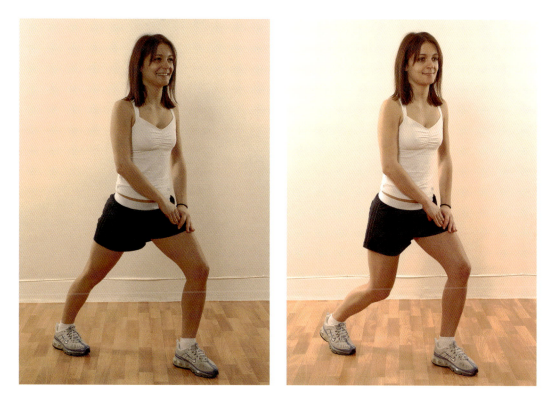

Lower leg – calf muscles

These muscles were not tested in chapter 2 because just about everyone has tight calves. Tightness in the calf muscles can limit the function of the foot and have a negative effect on movement, in particular running and walking. Almost everyone can benefit from stretching them out regularly, especially if you wear high heels.

- If necessary, start by leaning against a wall for support.
- Step back with one leg to a position where your heel is raised.
- Slowly and gently press your heel to the floor, feeling for the stretch in your lower leg.
- Hold for 30 seconds and repeat two to three times on each leg.

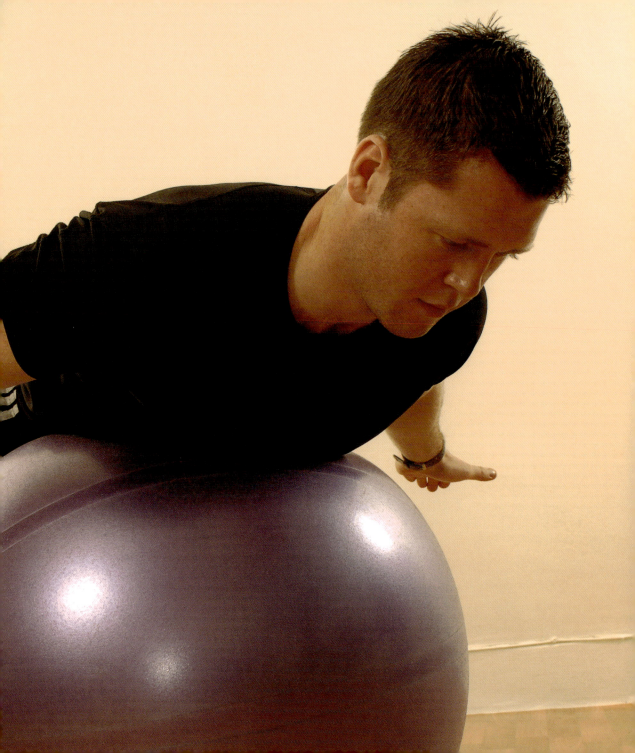

Core Stability – Developing Strength from Within

4

If there is one question personal trainers probably get asked more than any other, it's, 'How can I get a flat stomach?' Let's be honest, we would all love to have a set of those chiselled abdominals that are all over the covers of fitness magazines in your local newsagent's. This is the main reason why there are so many fad diets, fat loss pills, exercise machines, news articles and adverts that promise us the perfect beach body for very little effort. If you're thinking this sounds too good to be true, then you're right. The truth is that most, if not all, of these products are big on promises but fall a long way short on delivery. At best, they don't give us the results we want, while at worst they can actually increase our risk of injury, poor posture and back pain, leaving us with more problems than we started with.

The abdominal area has always been a hot topic, and more recently the trend has shifted towards training the 'core' of the body. Think about the way we move from day to day – getting out of a car, putting the bin out or swinging a golf club. These are all functional movements. But most abdominal training programmes do little to prepare our body for these movements; instead they focus on aesthetics and compromise function.

There is a lot more to training the abdominals than just looking good on the beach, although it is a nice bonus. The less glamorous side of abdominal training is about developing strength, and more importantly stability around the lower back and pelvis. Even fit and strong athletes can benefit from stability training. With over 80 per cent of us suffering from back pain at some stage in our lives, we can help prevent this debilitating problem and pre-empt future troubles. If your abdominals didn't test too well in chapter 2, or if you already suffer back pain, the exercises in this chapter are the ones for you.

THE LINK BETWEEN CORE STABILITY AND BACK PAIN

Back pain is the UK's leading cause of disability, with over 1.1 million people currently disabled by it. Around five million working days were lost to it in 2003 at a cost of around £150 million to the NHS. What makes this worse is that most back injuries are preventable, and yet they have still risen steadily over the past 10 years. Research shows a strong link between poorly working abdominals and lower back pain. In normal healthy people, the abdominal muscles spring into life which helps provide stability during movement. However, in people with back pain, these muscles don't function correctly, leaving them vulnerable to injury. Remember though, having a six-pack doesn't mean you won't suffer from back pain. When it comes to the lower back, train for *stability* instead of *mobility*.

It's not just about prevention either; by performing stability exercises, those who suffer from back problems can make real improvements in their function levels and reducing their pain. If you found the string tightening during the forward bending test in chapter 2, you could be at risk of problems, particularly if your daily life involves a lot of bending over (such as doing the gardening or moving furniture).

UNDERSTANDING HOW THE ABDOMINALS WORK

'Core stability' has been a fitness industry buzzword for some time now, so what does it actually mean? There are many excellent texts that detail the complex anatomy and biomechanics of the core in great detail, as well as many eminent researchers on the subject. However, the integrated nature of the core, involving muscles, fascia (the sheath that encases or often joins muscles), bones, organs, ligaments and tendons, is often confusing to the fitness professional, let alone the general public! So, let's try to highlight some of their key areas and functions, and look at why exactly core stability is so important.

As well as that six-pack muscle we know all about at the front of the torso, the core includes other muscles and organs, such as those in the lower back and sides that work together to provide strength and stability during movement. A strong and well-functioning core unit helps to provide a solid foundation for movements, such as pushing and pulling shown later in this book. Core stability also plays a big role in protecting the spine when we move and lift objects.

A popular way of explaining this is to think of the mid-section of the body as a cylinder that compresses its contents (in this case the spine and organs). As this happens, it increases the pressure inside the cylinder, making it stronger and more supportive of its contents. The clinical term for this is intra-abdominal pressure or IAP. This cylinder is formed by the abdominal and lumbar muscles on the sides, and at the top and bottom by the diaphragm and pelvic floor, respectively.

MUSCLE FACTS – THE PELVIC FLOOR

The muscles of the pelvic floor form the bottom of the cylinder that protects the spine during movement and lifting. Training these muscles is particularly valuable for pregnant women or those who suffer from incontinence. Better control of the pelvic floor muscles can also help improve your sex life (they help men to maintain an erection and women to have more intense sexual feelings).

To find your pelvic floor muscles, imagine trying to stop yourself while urinating. The muscles you can feel working deep inside are those of the pelvic floor. Learning to contract these in combination with the stabilising muscles can help increase stability and protect the pelvic organs.

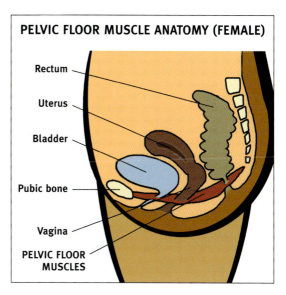

PELVIC FLOOR MUSCLE ANATOMY (FEMALE)

Rectum

Uterus

Bladder

Pubic bone

Vagina

PELVIC FLOOR MUSCLES

Though each of the abdominal muscles has a different job to do in the body, they do share some common roles. We can group them in two broad ways:

1 Movement muscles. Some of the core muscles have a major role in movement, such as bending, twisting or extending the trunk. These muscles tend to be closer to the surface and include the *rectus abdominis*, better known as the six-pack muscle.

2 Stabilising muscles. Beneath the more superficial core muscles lie those that help support and stabilise the spine and pelvis during movement. Often neglected by many training programmes, these muscles play an essential role in maintaining good back health and posture. These muscles tend to work at a lower level than our movement muscles and are

slower to tire. However, though they may have different individual roles, *all* our abdominal muscles play a very important role in supporting and protecting the spine during movement.

THE INTEGRATED AND ISOLATED FUNCTION OF THE CORE

It is important to remember that the body functions as one total unit. Although we can train areas such as the core in isolation, these muscles work together with the rest of the body to enable us to move and function better. Even when simply raising your arm to take a drink, the first muscles to work are those of the core. So, for our core training to be truly effective and functional, we should focus on combining the more static exercises that we use at the start with dynamic, multi-directional movement that will work the core as it is designed to be used, providing stability through motion.

An effective core-training programme needs to concentrate on the needs of both stabilising and movement muscles, and should not just be based on the sit-up or crunch movements. If your abs workout at the gym consists of 10 minutes spent on an ab-cradle or weighted sit-up machine at the end of the session, you need to change how you are training. Most fixed machines do little except help promote the hunched posture we saw in chapter 3. Despite this, people seem to be hypnotically drawn to them in the hope that a quick set of crunches will give them the eye-popping abs they want. Let me burst that bubble here and now, it won't! What it will do is develop muscle imbalance, poor posture and faulty movement patterns.

The exercises in this chapter help both stabilising and movement muscles, and will allow you to make a start towards balanced and effective core stability.

Remember that abdominal training should always begin by working on stability, *not* performance. Without proper control of the stabilising muscles, you can cause further problems and increase the risk of injury. Contrary to popular belief, it is *quality* that is important when training the core, not the *quantity*. By integrating the whole body movements shown later in this book with basic, simple core-specific movements, we can train the core to function correctly.

MUSCLE FACTS – THE TRANSVERSUS ABDOMINIS

The most commonly mentioned muscle when talking about core stability is the transversus abdominal muscle or TVA. As the name suggests, this muscle runs across our mid-section like a corset, and is the deepest of all the abdominal muscles. The function of the TVA has been the subject of a lot of debate among researchers on lower back problems, mostly with regard to how much it contributes to spinal stability. Rather than function independently, the TVA works with other muscles and tissues to provide stiffness and stability to the back. It is very hard to isolate the action of TVA, so rather than trying to concentrate on a specific muscle, simply learning to activate the abdominals can help maintain good core positioning during exercise. Remember that these muscles work at a lower intensity, and you shouldn't be squeezing too hard, as

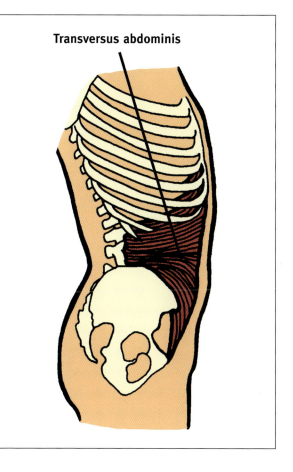

Transversus abdominis

this can cause the upper back to flex forwards, which is incorrect. You should be able to breathe normally when practising this. It is natural to hold the breath when lifting a heavy object, but this can cause dangerous rises in blood pressure and should not be practised during the exercises in this book. Learning to activate the abdominals should help retrain them to work more effectively, and will become automatic over time.

Pelvic positioning – neutral position

Getting the pelvis in the right position during exercise can be challenging, as it takes time to develop a good level of awareness in this area. Put simply, you are trying to avoid positions where you are arching or flexing your lower back excessively. A 'neutral' spine is often the word used to describe the ideal pelvic position. Pelvic rocks are a simple way to find and practise pelvic positioning.

- Stand with your hands at your waist just above the pelvis.
- Roll your pelvis forwards, feeling your lower back arch.
- Gently roll the pelvis back, flattening your lower back. When you do this, it is really important to maintain good posture in the trunk and not to bend forwards (which will be the tendency).

The neutral spine position is midway between the two extremes of pelvic movement and is the starting point for all your exercises. It is a good idea to start your workouts with this movement until you feel practised at it.

Core training provides us with strength from within. It enables us to develop strength, speed and power (all necessary for movement) without compromising the spine and pelvis. It is necessary for us all to include core training as part of a successful training programme, so if you're ready to get started, let's go! Remember, as with all the exercises in this book, they have to be done correctly to be effective – follow the guidelines below and use the photographs to help.

FIVE TIPS FOR SUCCESSFUL ABDOMINAL TRAINING

1 You can get too much of a good thing, and exercise is no different. So you can do 1000 crunches? So what? When it comes to working out, it is quality over quantity that gets results. This is especially true where the core is concerned, so focus on good technique and quality of movement over the numbers and results will come.

2 Steer clear of sit-ups. Though there is a time and place for sit-ups in abdominal training, they favour the muscles of the hip rather than the stomach and are often done incorrectly, causing more harm than good. At best you'll be wasting workout time; at worst you'll be

subjecting your lower back to high levels of stress over and over again. The only person who will benefit from this is your osteopath or chiropractor!

3 Give the core time to recover from a workout. Like any other muscle, the abdominals can be overtrained. Only train core muscles three to four times a week.

4 For those just starting to exercise, I recommend training the core at the start of a workout. The chances are that your technique and application will be best at the start of a session. As you progress, core training will become more integrated into your main routine and will become more dynamic. It can be hard to maintain motivation to do stability training, so regularly change your exercises and when you do them to add variety to the workout.

5 Focus on quality over quantity. Don't compromise your form to squeeze out that last repetition. Once the abdominals have started to fail, they have been overloaded and that's good enough.

ABDOMINAL ACTIVATION

Before we begin to do anything else, we need to learn how to contract our deep abdominal muscles. This action helps us to maintain stability and support around the spine, whatever we are doing, and it is important to master it before moving onto more dynamic exercises.

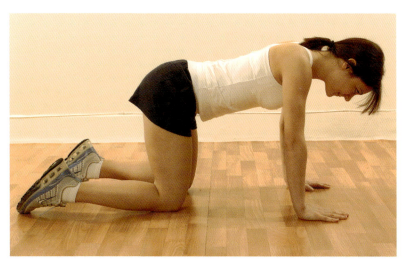

This simple exercise can greatly improve stability of the lower back and strengthen the deep abdominal muscles.

■ Start on all fours with your hips over your knees and your shoulders directly over your hands.

- Feel the abdominals tense but don't try to suck them inwards.

- For day-to-day life, low levels of actual muscle activation are needed. You should feel a gentle contraction.

- Maintain a normal breathing pattern, which you should be able to do under low levels of load.

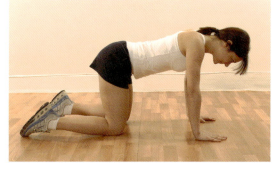

- Hold this position for 10 seconds, relax and repeat 10 times.

Too easy?

Once you have mastered this exercise on all fours, you can progress to perform it in kneeling and in standing positions.

Too hard?

If you find this exercise too difficult on all fours or if you have any kind of wrist or knee injury that may be made worse, try the exercise lying on your back.

Note: Getting the pelvis in the right position during core work can be tricky. The ideal is to aim for a neutral position as shown in chapter 3. This means that there should be a slight arch in the lower back.

LEG LOCK FLOOR BRIDGE

The floor bridge is an excellent exercise to strengthen the muscles of the backside. By locking the leg into the body it prevents the lower back from arching, which is a common fault when performing this exercise.

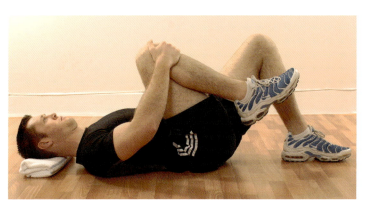

- Lie on your back on the floor.

- Bring one leg into your chest and hold it there.

Keep the other leg bent with the foot flat on the floor.

- Activating the abdominals, squeeze your bum and lift your backside off the floor between 3in and 6in.

- Hold at the top of the movement and control the return back to the floor.

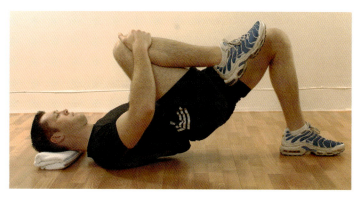

Too easy?

If you find this exercise easy, it sounds like your hip muscles are working well. Increase the challenge by holding at the top of the movement for five seconds on each repetition. Alternatively, try the exercise with the feet on a stability ball.

Too hard?

If this is proving too difficult, reduce the intensity by placing both your feet on the floor and doing a bridge from that position. Take care to keep your belly button drawn in and not to let your lower back arch.

LOWER ABS BLASTER

This is a great exercise for challenging the lower abdominal area. Remember, good form is really important, so be sure *not* to let your lower back arch when performing this exercise.

- Lie on your back on the floor with your hips and knees bent to 90 degrees.

- Find and maintain a neutral spine position throughout the movement.

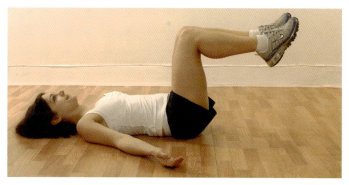

- Slowly lower one leg towards the floor without letting your lower back arch and rise off the floor. Don't let your foot touch the floor.

- Return to the start position, then repeat on the other leg.

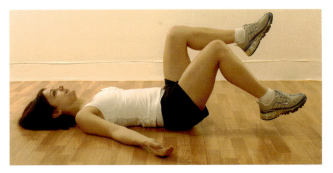

Too easy?

If you find this exercise easy, it sounds like your abdominals are working well. Increase the challenge by lowering both legs together.

Too hard?

If this is proving too difficult, try not to lower your legs as far towards the floor. Even with a shorter range of movement you will still feel the benefits of this exercise.

OPPOSITE ARM AND LEG RAISE

This movement is another stability-focused exercise. This time, by raising opposite limbs, it challenges the rotational muscles of the core to stabilise and prevent movement. This is an ideal exercise for those starting out on their training, or a great core warm-up for those more practised.

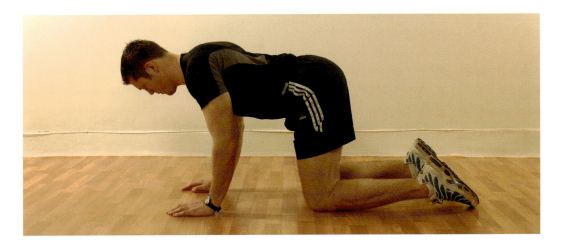

- Begin in the same position as for the abdominal activation exercise.

- Maintaining the position, raise one arm forwards and to the side, while at the same time extending the opposite leg away from your body.

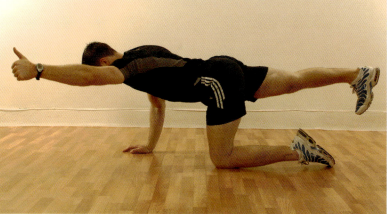

- Return to the start position, then repeat on the opposite side.

To do this movement correctly, your pelvis should remain level and not tilt from side to side as the leg lifts. To check this isn't happening, place a book on your lower back as you do the exercise. If it slides off, you are tilting your hips and you need to begin with the simpler version shown below.

Too easy?

If this feels easy, try performing the exercise over a stability ball; select a small ball for this. It will add an extra challenge to your stability.

Too hard?

If this is proving too difficult, start off by only raising your arms, keeping your feet on the floor. Once you have mastered this, progress to raising your knee off the floor but keep your toes down. Then you'll be ready to progress to the full version shown above.

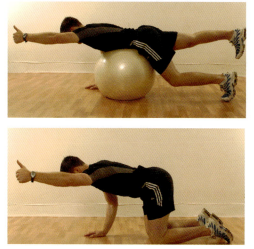

THE PLANK

This is one exercise that is all too often performed badly. Remember, for the exercise to be effective, it must be done correctly. Follow the guidelines below and you should feel your abdominal muscles working hard to hold the position.

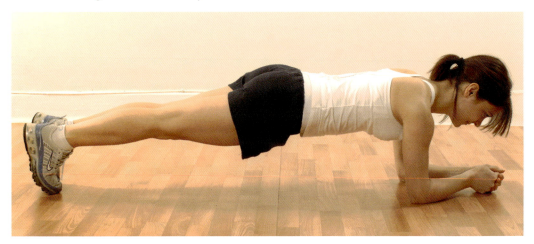

- Start with your forearms on the floor and your elbows slightly behind the shoulders.
- Tuck your toes under and lift your body off the floor.
- Activate your abdominals and squeeze your bum.
- Take care not to let your lower back arch or your upper back round during this exercise.

Too easy?

If you are able to hold this position with good form for a minute, you can increase the challenge by adding alternate leg-lifting. Perform these by squeezing your bum and lifting your leg 6in from the floor. Ensure that you keep your belly button drawn in when doing this.

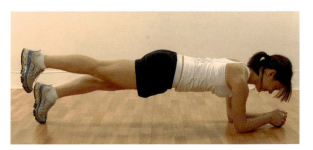

Too hard?

Done right, this is a hard exercise. To reduce the intensity slightly, perform the exercise as above, except with your knees on the floor.

PRONE COBRA

This core exercise targets the muscles

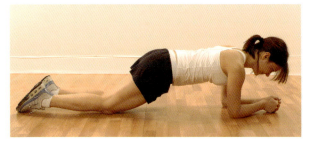

of the mid- and lower back, buttocks and core, and is a great exercise for improving posture. As this exercise has a strong postural focus, it works best when the position is held over time.

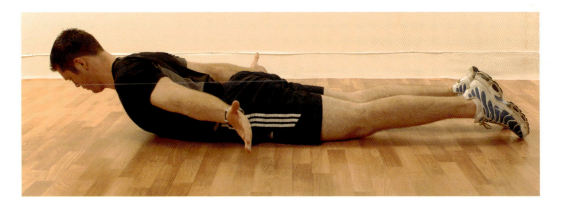

- Lying on the floor, tighten the muscles of the bum (glutes).

- Keep your chin tucked in and look towards the floor during the exercise. Resist the temptation to look up, extending the neck.

- Raise your chest off the floor and lift your arms, rotating your thumbs towards the ceiling.

- Hold at the top of the movement, and be sure not to lift up too high and excessively arch your lower back.

Too easy?

Try performing this exercise on a stability ball, but not until you can hold it for a minute on the floor!

Too hard?

Start with short holds and try to gradually increase the amount of time you can hold the position.

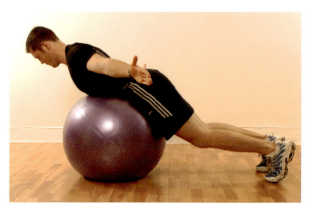

RUSSIAN TWISTS

The Russian twist exercise targets the rotational muscles of the core. These muscles provide movement and stability during nearly all activities of daily life, particularly during sports such as golf, tennis, squash and running.

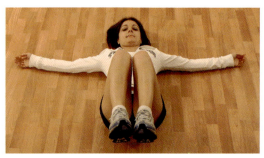

- Lie on your back on the floor with your hips and knees bent to 90 degrees.
- Slowly lower your legs together to one side.
- Return to the start position, then repeat on the opposite side.

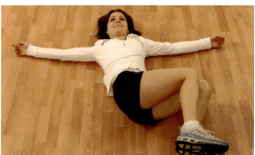

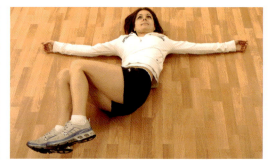

Too easy?

If you find this exercise too easy, increase the intensity by straightening your legs.

Too hard?

If this is proving too difficult, try not to lower your legs as far towards the floor. Even with a shorter range of movement, you will still feel the benefits of this exercise. Alternatively, reduce the challenge by placing the feet on a stability ball.

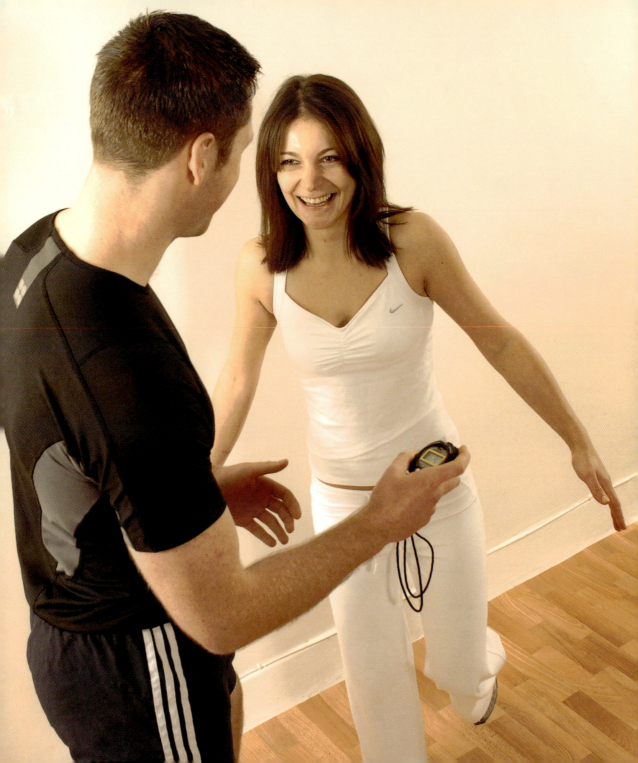

Better Balance

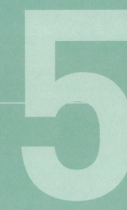

Balance training is an important part of any training programme, as it is the ability to balance that keeps us upright when we walk, play sport and perform everyday jobs and activities. But it is a skill that is all too often taken for granted, and is a neglected aspect of many training programmes. Very few fitness machines or common weights routines challenge our balance; many actually remove the need to balance in order to lift more weight. Now, this is a fairly sensible course of action if you are planning to squat 300kg, but if you want a programme that covers all aspects of your fitness, balance training must be part of it.

As we age, our ability to balance starts to get worse. Part of the reason for this are changes in the systems within our muscles that convey vital information to our brain about posture and movement. This loss of balance increases the risk of injury from falling and can impair performance in work, home life and sport.

But it is not just as we age that balance becomes important. For many active jobs and sports, good balance is essential. Think about the ability of a rugby player to sidestep an opponent, an ice skater to perform movements, or a firefighter who needs to be able to move in dark and difficult conditions. To all these people, balance plays an integral part in what they do.

By improving our balance, we develop a better sense of movement, coordination and perception. This can help to prevent falls, improve posture, and help improve confidence and stability.

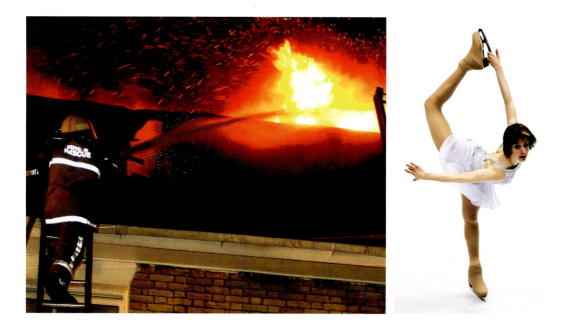

SO HOW EXACTLY DO WE STAY IN BALANCE?

The body maintains balance through a number of different ways. Three systems work together to help us stay on two feet.

1 Visual

2 Sensory

3 Vestibular (in the inner ear)

Each system supplies the brain with valuable information on movement, position, orientation and our surroundings, which it then converts into messages for our muscles to adapt to. All these systems can be affected by age, environment, illness or injury. Any disruption to one system can have a significant effect on how we move and function, although the other systems will often learn to adjust and compensate for this.

We rely on these three systems to generate information that helps us maintain balance. Sight may be an obvious thing that we rely on to balance – but think back to the single leg balance test in chapter 2! What we see tells us a lot about our head and neck position, as well as what's going on around us. We also get a tremendous amount of information from something in our muscles and joints known as *proprioceptors*. These tiny sensors send back information to the brain about joint position, and changes in the length and tension of the muscles, helping regulate posture and movement.

Finally, our balance is also aided by the structure of the inner ear. Fluid and small hairs inside the ear send messages back to the brain about head movement and acceleration. Each system is vulnerable to changes from age or injury but can also be significantly improved with training.

Proprioceptors in action

The body is an incredibly clever thing – have you ever wondered how, even with your eyes closed, you can tell if you are seated or standing, or know if an arm is bent or straight? Without us realising it, proprioceptors in the body are constantly feeding back information that allows the body to adjust to its surroundings. This is how a high-diver is able to know their position in space as they head towards the water. For most of us, though, it means that, through developing an awareness of our movement, we can greatly improve our balance and agility.

CAUSES OF BALANCE PROBLEMS

There are three main reasons why balance can become poor.

1 Injury: If we injure any area that is linked to our ability to balance (eyes, inner ear, spinal cord), it affects how we process and deliver information to and from the muscles. Similarly, if you injure a part of your body, such as badly spraining your ankle, this can lead to damage to those sensors or proprioceptors around the joint. The same effect has been seen in people with knee and hip problems. This has been strongly linked by research into decreased ability to balance.

2 Illness: Illness can also affect our ability to balance effectively; an example of this that many of us have experienced is an ear infection. This can cause vertigo (a feeling of spinning or falling) even when perfectly stable. More serious conditions such as Parkinson's disease or Huntington's disease also negatively affect the ability to balance.

3 Ageing: Ageing is probably the most prevalent factor leading to poorer balance. With the loss of strength and power that comes with inactivity, there is a significant decrease in the ability to maintain balance successfully. Many elderly people also fear falling; this fear is associated with poor health, low functional ability, depression, anxiety, and a low quality of life. Clearly, balance training should be an important aspect of all fitness programmes that aim to improve quality of life.

Ankle sprains and balance training

One of the most common injuries people suffer is a sprained ankle. These are normally when the ankle is 'turned over', causing damage to the tissue around the joint. This often causes severe bruising, pain and instability. The feeling of instability can last for years after the injury, and is one of the reasons why the injury is likely to be repeated on the same leg in the future. This injury can also lead to a change in how muscles work at the hip, leading to muscle imbalance and further problems.

Balance training can help regain the stability on injured ankles and should form part of any recovery regime. By improving our proprioceptors, we can begin to increase stability and restore normal muscle function, essential for a full recovery.

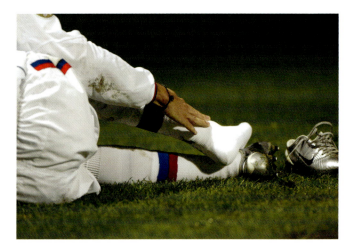

HOW CAN TRAINING IMPROVE BALANCE?

Almost all the exercises shown in this book will have a positive effect on improving balance. This is due to the wide range of influences that can affect our ability to stay balanced; these include posture, muscle tightness or weakness, awareness of the body in movement (also known as kinaesthetic awareness), and the ability of the lower body to generate strength and power.

Ninety per cent of hip fractures result from a fall. In 2001, nearly 70,000 people in the UK were injured when falling over. Home-based exercise programmes that include low-intensity strength and balance training have improved balance and reduced fall rates by around 40 per cent, compared to controls. One study showed improvements in balance equivalent to someone three to 10 years younger, by training simply three times a week.

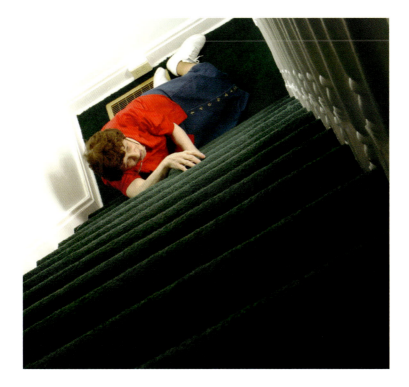

It is important to develop your balance training from the simpler exercises first, before attempting the more complex ones. The focus should be on working at the threshold of function, *not* failure. If you find yourself constantly losing balance while doing the exercise, try a slightly easier version first.

When training to improve balance, the goal is to try to maintain the centre of gravity of the body over its base. As we develop the optimal ways in which to do this, these patterns of movement start to become automatic. This allows the body to begin to predict a loss of balance and get the muscles working in preparation to prevent falls and to increase stability.

Each of the exercises shown is designed specifically to improve this skill, along with options to increase or decrease the challenge, as needed. So, if you're ready, let's get started!

MAKING AN ARCH

Before we get too far with the various balance exercises, it is important to get the muscles of the foot working right first. The arch of the foot is critical for absorbing shock efficiently, and is full of sensors that give us the valuable information that can help with movement and balance. Many problems are caused in the body by the feet not working the way they should. This can cause pain in the base of the foot, but also further up in the knee, hip and lower back. To form an arch in the foot, you'll need to be barefoot.

- Gently lift your big toe upwards towards your head; you will feel your weight shift slightly to the outside of your foot. You should also feel the arch of the foot form. Feel for the muscles in your foot that are maintaining the arch and try not to curl all your other toes up.

- Without losing the arch in your foot, slowly relax your big toe back down towards the floor.

The muscles you felt working help to control movement of the foot during static exercises and also during walking and running. This does take a bit of practice, so, if you need to, begin in a seated position before progressing to standing and then onto balancing.

Note: Perform all your balance training without your shoes on. This will help to improve the feeling and sensation in your feet, making them more sensitive to what is happening underneath them.

SINGLE LEG BALANCE – BASIC

The single leg balance is the starting point for the balance exercises. It helps develop stability and feeling through the foot and ankle, as well as strengthening the muscles of the supporting hip.

- Start by making an arch in the supporting foot.

- Lift one leg off the floor, bringing your knee forwards slightly, keeping your foot relaxed.

- Ensure that your knee stays over the second/third toes and that your hips, knees and shoulders stay level during the exercise.

Initially, start this exercise with your eyes open. Once you can balance for a minute with them open, progress to trying it with them closed.

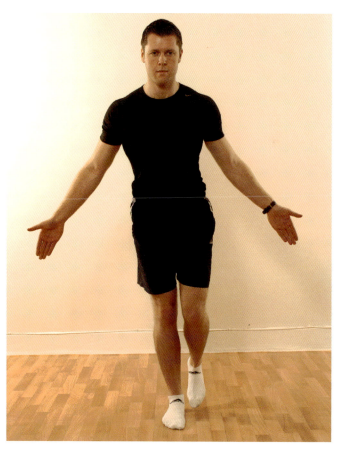

CLOCKFACE REACHES

The next progression from a single leg balance exercise is to add reaching movements with the free leg. Reaching movements challenge the body to stay in balance through all

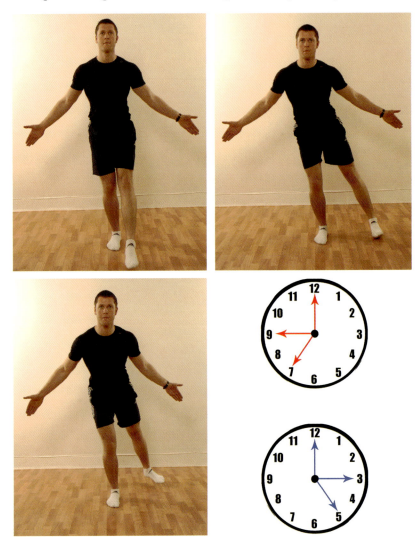

planes of movement, improve stability and coordination, and encourage movement at the ankle joint.

■ Start as for a single leg balance exercise.

■ This time move the free leg forwards, out to the side, then diagonally back and out.

■ Imagine a clockface on the floor under your supporting leg. Aim to reach for 12, then 3 – or 9 depending which leg you are standing on – and then either 5 or 7.

■ Aim to reach as far as possible without losing your balance.

■ Ensure that you keep your knee, hip and shoulders all level.

TOUCHDOWNS

The touchdown exercise is more dynamic and challenging. This total-body balancing exercise will also improve leg and hip strength, as well as dynamic balance. Remember, stay within your limits; if at first you find the full range of movement difficult, work with a shorter range, which will make the exercise easier.

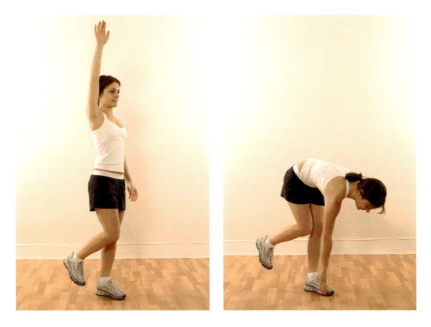

- Start with the single leg stance and a good arch in your foot.
- Raise your arm (same side as the free leg) overhead and slowly lower it, reaching down to touch your toes.
- Keep your free leg next to the supporting leg.
- Feel the muscles of your bum work as you stand back up.

LUNGE TO KNEE RAISE

The lunge to balance movement is a difficult and complex one that really challenges the body to balance dynamically. It is a great exercise to improve strength in the hips and thighs; it also challenges the core muscles to help maintain a stable posture throughout.

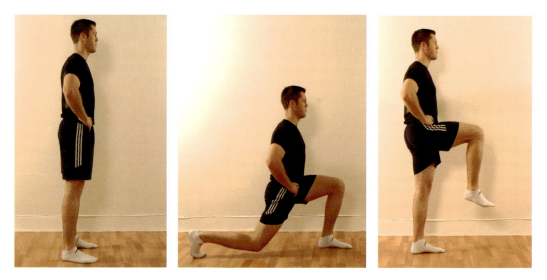

- Start with feet parallel and hip-width apart. Place your hands on your hips.
- Take a good step backwards, keeping your feet at hip-distance apart.
- Lower your hips towards the floor, keeping the rear knee just off the ground.
- Bring the knee forwards and upwards into a single leg balance.
- Place your foot down and repeat on the other leg.

HOP, STOP AND GO

The hop and stop exercise helps to improve dynamic balance in all three planes of movement. It incorporates reflex movements with the ability to move quickly from one foot to another. This exercise will help to improve sports performance and will allow you to regain balance where before it might have led to a fall. Begin this exercise working simply forwards and backwards, then introduce the lateral and rotational movements as soon as possible.

■ Start with your feet hip-width apart and looking straight ahead.

■ Hop forward and bring your knee up into a balance position.

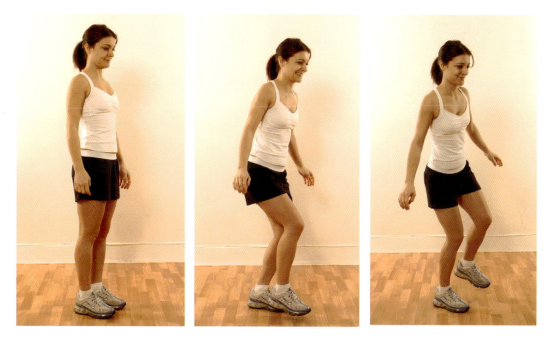

■ Hold the position for a count of two, then hop back to the start and repeat on the other leg.

■ Perform the movement forwards and backwards, to the side and back, and finally, diagonally backwards.

■ As you improve, aim to increase the distance you hop, along with the speed.

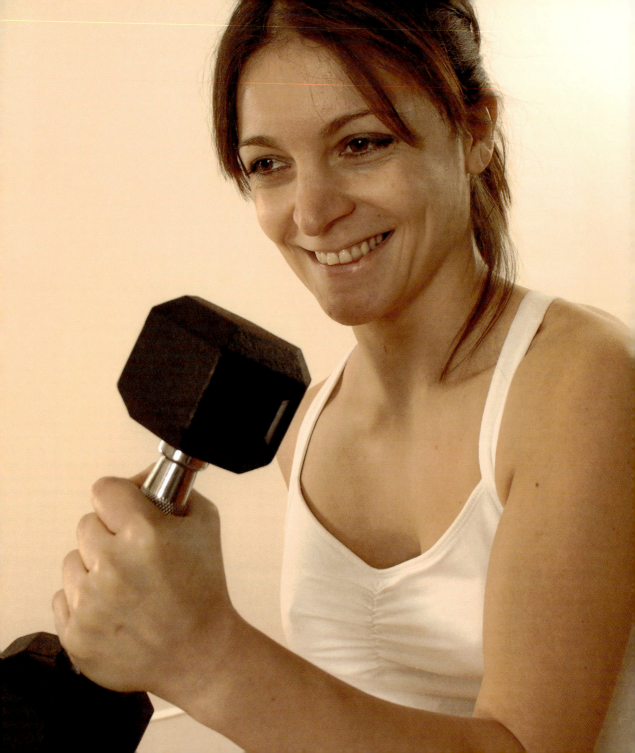

Movement-Based Resistance Training (MBRT) – Developing Functional Fitness

6

Now we have covered the fundamentals of mobility, stability and balance, we are ready to really get moving! In this section, we will look at how we can use movement and resistance to increase strength, power, balance, coordination and agility. Using a range of exercises designed to challenge the body through each plane of movement, this section will improve your ability to perform everyday activities. The human body thinks and works in movements, not by individual muscles. Traditional approaches have favoured programmes to train separate muscle groups, such as the chest, back and shoulders, instead of training the patterns of movement that we use in everyday life. Fixed-resistance machines found in health clubs are not geared towards improving how we function. They generally require you to sit or lie down, and rob the body of the need to stabilise itself during the exercise, something it simply must do in real life. Sitting down also increases load through the spine and discs, which, when combined with poor technique or high loads, can be potentially dangerous. In short, they are bad news for most of us!

Although there are those who may benefit from using machines, most people are better off working with freeweights and just their bodyweight in an environment that challenges the whole body in all planes of movement. This approach forms the basis of what I call movement-based resistance training (MBRT).

Rather than divide the body by muscles, we will be training it by the following movements:

Squatting and bending

Pushing

Pulling

Lunging and stepping

By recreating movements that we use every day, we can develop strength, coordination, balance and power that transfers into everything we do, whether it is work, sport or simply carrying the shopping home. These movements make us use our bodyweight over added weight. You have to carry your bodyweight around with you all day, so why not train to be able to do this better? As we have already seen, strength without stability is useless in the real world. First, learn to support your own weight, and then start adding weight.

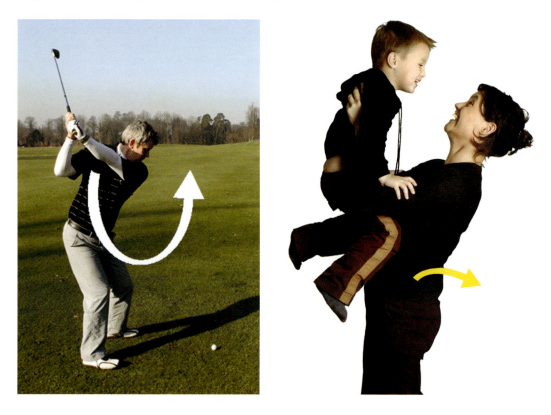

TRAINING WITH A TWIST

Human movements are never purely two-dimensional; whatever we do involves some amount of bending, extending, twisting and lateral movement. Think about a movement such as getting in and out of a car, and how we have to squat, step, twist, bend, push and pull to do it. Many exercise programmes and gym machines favour movements forwards and backwards, but rarely do they incorporate twisting, stepping, or bending into those movements to make them truly functional (see right).

By moving in different directions and planes, we get a better crossover to everyday life and can add interest and challenge to our workouts.

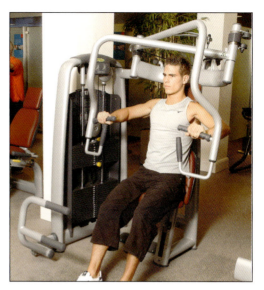

Get more bang for your buck!

Exercise machines just can't give us the same kind of workout that we can get from movement-based training. It would take you at least four machines to equal the effect of a squat or lunging exercise. So, to save time, money and waiting in line for your machine at the gym, stick to free weights and movement-based exercises such as those in this chapter.

MBRT allows greater flexibility of training, addresses a wide range of training outcomes and can be done just about anywhere with a minimum of equipment. However, some of the exercises do require a little equipment to perform, which you can either buy or hire in your local gym or sports centre.

Many of the exercises shown use your own bodyweight for resistance, but, particularly during *pulling* movements, this can be difficult to do. For that reason, I recommend either obtaining a set of adjustable dumbbells if possible (something like the Sportblock is ideal and sells for around £100) or simply using exercise bands or tubing, which are considerably cheaper (around £10–£20 for a set). These come in various weights for different exercises and are simple to use, portable and easy to store; they are an excellent option for home-based training or working out on the move.

SQUATTING AND BENDING

There isn't a day that goes by when you won't have to squat or bend at some point. Sometimes, it might be just to sit on or stand up from a chair, pick up your shoes, or perhaps something else as part of your job. These movements develop strength and stability around the ankle, knee and hip joints. A lack of strength around these joints can contribute to poor balance and stability, difficulty with everyday tasks, added wear and tear on joints, and fatigue during activity.

As well as having excellent health benefits, the exercises shown here will also strengthen, tighten and tone the muscle around your buttocks and thighs, improving your body shape.

The squat is one of the most functional and versatile movements that you can do. It is used by everyone from bodybuilders trying to get bigger legs to physiotherapists dealing with rehabilitation of the lower body. It is sometimes referred to as the 'king' of all resistance training exercises, not only for its wide range of applications, but also for the large amount of muscle you use when performing it.

Basic squat

The basic squat movement is one of the most functional movement patterns that we use every day. This is the basic variation of the exercise. If you find it difficult to maintain form on this, use a stability ball behind you to create extra support.

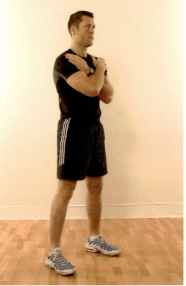

- Start with your feet a comfortable distance apart, slightly wider than shoulder-width.

- Your arms can be folded across your chest or held out to the front.

- Bend at the hips, knees and ankle as if sitting on a chair.

- Keep your knees over your toes and lower your body towards the floor.

■ Return to the start position by extending through your knees and hips.

Note: Squat depth – how far down you should squat – is a contentious issue among fitness professionals. Many texts wrongly suggest that squatting beyond a point where your thighs are parallel with the floor is dangerous, but this is not always true. You should squat as far down as you can while maintaining good form. For most people (particularly when starting out), this is around the point at which the thighs are parallel with the floor. If you suffer from knee pain, use a shorter, pain-free, range of movement.

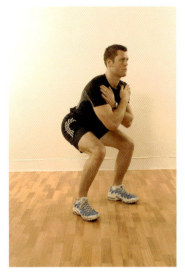

Split stance squat

The split stance squat is an excellent alternative to the basic squat. This simple exercise really mimics how we stand to lift and move objects, and develops real functional strength in the legs and hips.

■ Start by taking a short stride forward, keeping your feet shoulder-width apart.

■ Bend through your knees and ankles, lowering your hips to the floor, keeping your trunk upright.

■ Extend through your knees and ankles back to the start position.

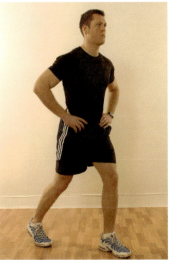
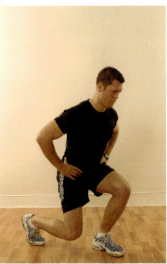

Overhead squat

This is one exercise that is a lot harder to do than it looks. Not only does it develop great leg strength, but it also helps to improve core strength and shoulder mobility. You can use a piece of rubber tubing or simply a towel to do this exercise.

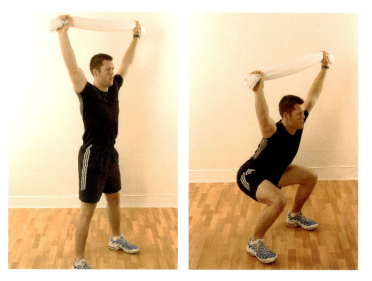

- Start as for the basic squat.

- Raise your arms straight overhead, keeping the towel or tubing held tightly between them.

- Squat, keeping your arms directly overhead; avoid arching your back or allowing your arms to fall forward.

- Keep good alignment of your knees over your toes; only go down as far as you can while keeping excellent form.

Bulgarian squat

The Bulgarian-style squat really challenges the muscles at the front of the thigh and, as well as building strength, it is an excellent move for improving stability around the knee joint.

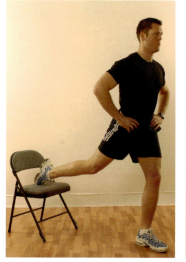

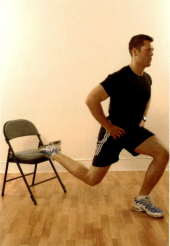

- Take a good-sized stride forwards, keeping your feet shoulder-width apart.

- Place your rear foot onto a step (or you can use a chair or low table).

- Keeping your hands at your hips and your trunk upright, lower your hips towards the floor.

- Keep your knee in good alignment over your toes.

Single leg squat – arms out to front

Not an exercise for the faint-hearted, the single leg squat is one of the most challenging bodyweight exercises you can do for the legs. This exercise can help build strength throughout the whole body and really challenges the muscles that stabilise the body during movement.

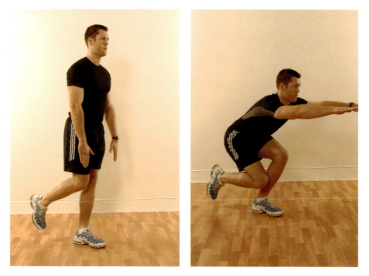

- Stand on one leg, with the raised leg bent at the knee and ankle, and held next to the supporting leg throughout the movement.

- Squat, bending at the hip, knee and ankle. Only go as far as possible, keeping good form.

- Ensure your knee doesn't collapse and that it remains over your toes.

- Extend through your knee and hips back to the start position.

PUSHING

Pushing and pulling movements target the muscles of the upper extremity and core. They are often performed in daily life with a lower-extremity movement such as walking, squatting, lunging or bending. They also often involve twisting movements, which means that good core strength and coordination are really important when you are doing these exercises. This kind of pattern in how we move further reminds us of the importance of integrated movement in our training, which has a high level of crossover with how we live and move from day to day.

Balanced strength through these movements will develop the muscles around the shoulders and chest, as well as the back and arms. Pulling movements can be difficult to perform with only bodyweight, so many of the exercises in this chapter are shown using simple pieces of equipment such as exercise bands and tubing or dumbbells.

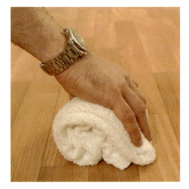

Note: Pushing exercises can be stressful on the wrist joints. If you suffer from a wrist-related injury or condition such as arthritis, use a small towel or similar item to reduce the amount of wrist extension needed for these exercises. People can often compromise their core stability during pushing exercises, so make sure you keep excellent form and perform the essential stretches for any tight areas before you start.

Wall push-up

The wall push-up is a simple introduction to pushing movements. It is an ideal exercise to help improve stability around the shoulders and core, and will strengthen the chest, shoulders and arms ready for more demanding versions. Ensure that the floor surface is not slippery and try not to leave any handprints on your wall!

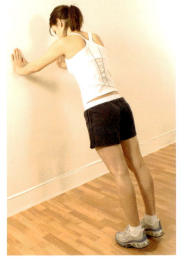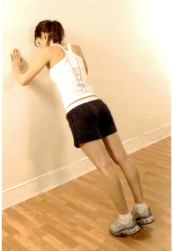

- Stand with your feet around a metre from the wall.

- Extend your arms and lean forwards, placing them against the wall.

- Bend your elbows, allowing your chest to move towards the wall.

- Avoid bending at the hips; keep the core strong and your body in good alignment.
- Extend your arms back to the start position.

Fitball press-up

Using a stability ball can really help make the transition to a full press-up, as it helps shorten the lever length of the body. If you don't have a stability ball, you can do a press-up from the knees, although this isn't as effective for developing the core strength needed for a full press-up.

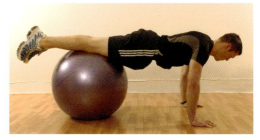

- Begin with your thighs resting on the ball.
- Bend your elbows, lowering your body to 90 degrees.
- Extend back to the start position.
- The further you move from the ball, the harder the exercise.

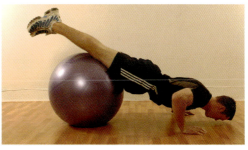

Press-up

The full press-up movement is a total body exercise that requires strength, not only in the movement muscles of the chest, shoulders, and arms, but also a great deal of core strength to maintain good form.

Only perform this exercise if you are able to perform the plank exercise shown in chapter 3.

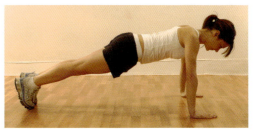

- Start with your toes tucked under and arms extended, ensuring your whole body is in good alignment. You should be able to hold this position without rounding your upper back, arching your lower back or lifting your hips.

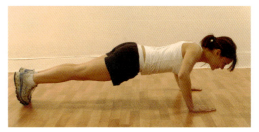

■ Bend your elbows and lower your whole body towards the floor, maintaining perfect body alignment.

■ Extend through your chest and arms to return to the start position.

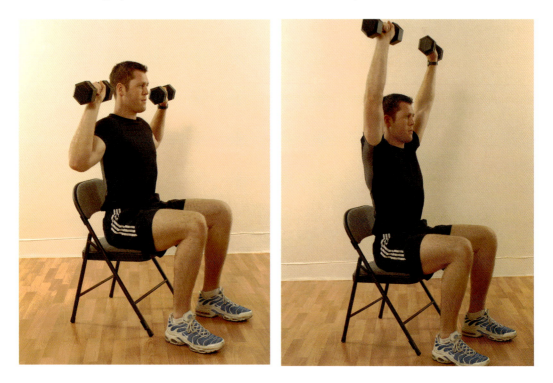

Overhead press – seated

This exercise builds strength by working above the head, and helps to shape and develop the muscles of the shoulder. The common mistake with this exercise is to compromise form to achieve the weight. Don't make that mistake; keep the core muscles working to prevent arching your lower back excessively, as this transfers high loads to the spine.

■ Sit either on a chair or a stability ball.

■ Using either dumbbells or tubing, start with your arms at shoulder height and palms facing away.

- Keeping your back in good alignment, press your arms overhead.

- If you find this hard to do without arching your back, then try the single-arm standing version shown below.

- Keeping the movement under control, lower your arms back to the start position.

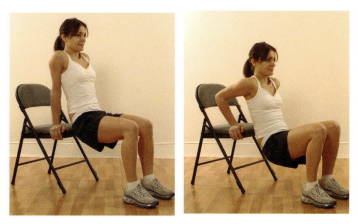

Dips

Dips are not only a classic exercise, but also a functional movement for building strength in the upper arms and shoulders. This movement is commonly used when rising or sitting, or when pushing up from something. Increase the challenge by moving your feet further from your body when you perform the exercise.

- Begin with the knees and hips bent to 90 degrees in a seated position.

- Place your hands on the edge of a chair, bench or solid surface.

- Lower your body till your arms are bent to around 90 degrees.

- Extend back to the start position.

Single-arm overhead press – standing

This is an ideal way to improve strength in your shoulder area for lifting overhead. Performing the single-arm movement allows the body to rotate, protecting the lumbar spine from injury.

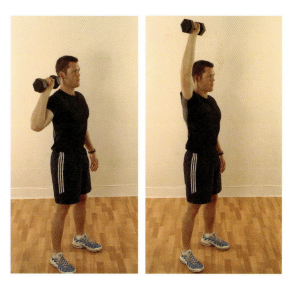

- Stand with your feet shoulder-width apart.
- Using either dumbbells, tubing or improvised weights, press one arm overhead.
- Allow movement at your knee and hip; this is functional and has a better crossover with real life.
- Alternate sides.

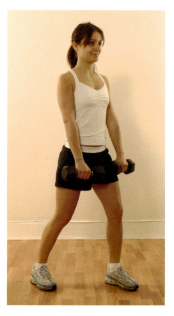

PULLING

Bodyweight pulling movements are among the most challenging exercises around. So, to develop better strength and stability in this movement pattern, you will need to use some resistance instead of your own bodyweight.

High pulls

The high pull exercise targets muscles in the shoulder and arms, as well as building core strength for many everyday tasks. For this (as with most pulling movements), you will need to use something other than bodyweight to create resistance. This can be tubing or dumbbells, or you can improvise with a weighted bag or box, for example.

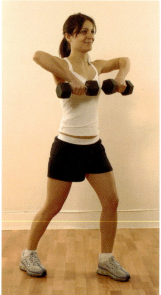

- Start with your feet slightly wider than shoulder-width apart (a split stance can be used if preferred).
- Hold the weights/tubing to the front.
- Draw your elbows towards the ceiling, keeping the resistance close to your body.
- Keep increasing the resistance as far as your chest, then return to the start position under control.
- Ensure your lower back does not arch and that your chin does not protrude forwards.

Bent-over pull

The bent-over row/pull is a staple exercise for weightlifters and athletes everywhere. As well as developing strength in the pulling muscles of the back, it also challenges core strength and posture by working the lower back and buttocks to hold the exercise position. It's a must-do exercise for total body strength.

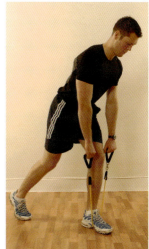

- Start with your feet slightly wider than shoulder-width apart.

- Bend forwards from your hips, ensuring that you keep a slight arch in your lower back.

- Look ahead – relaxing your neck muscles also causes your lower back muscles to relax.

- Keep the resistance close to your body throughout the movement.

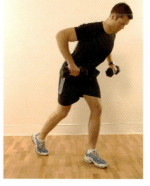

- Using a wide grip, pull the resistance in towards your abdomen. Take care to maintain good posture while doing this.

- Control the weight back to the start position.

Pullovers

Pullovers can either be done lying on a bench, step or, best of all, a stability ball. This movement will help stretch tight muscles of the chest and back actively, while also challenging core muscles to maintain correct pelvic positioning.

The tendency with this exercise is to arch your lower back, so prevent this by focusing on keeping your abdominals tight and your backside tightly squeezed.

- Sit on the stability ball or bench. Move into a supine position. If using a ball, ensure that your head and shoulders are supported.

- Hold the weights overhead with your arms extended straight up towards the ceiling.

- Keeping a slight bend at your elbow, slowly lower your arms behind your head. Make sure you do not arch your lower back.

- Return to the start position.

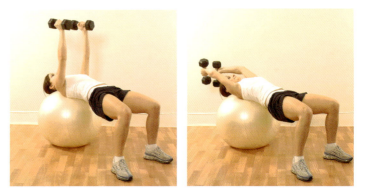

Archer's pull

For this exercise you will need a piece of tubing or resistance band. One of my favourite movements, the archer's pull emulates truly lifelike patterns by combining the actions of pulling and twisting. This means that you are training the muscles of your back along with those of the core that control rotation.

- Start in a split stance with the opposite leg forward to the arm which is pulling.

- Keep your free arm held high to maintain good shoulder alignment.

- Draw back your arm as if you were drawing back the string of a bow.

- Allow your shoulders to rotate back so that your body twists with the movement (this should come from the upper back, *not* the lower back).

- Return the arm under control.

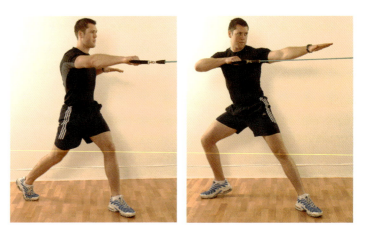

Uppercuts

Another one of my favourite exercises, the uppercut again combines the muscles of the shoulders and back with those of the core. It helps to train dynamic movement between the pelvis and spine, as well as developing powerful arms and shoulders. You can either use dumbbells or improvised weights for this movement.

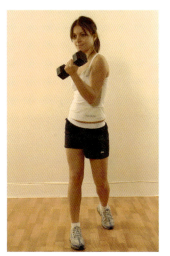

- Start with your feet around shoulder-width apart.

- Turning your palm towards your chest, rotate your body to one side and perform an uppercut movement, bending at the elbow and shoulder. Allow your hips and feet to twist with your upper body.

- Return to the start position and perform on the opposite side.

LUNGING AND STEPPING

These movements have a very strong crossover with one of the most important areas of human movement, known as gait. Gait is the term that refers to movements on foot such as walking, jogging or running. Just as when we walk or run, lunging and stepping are exercises where the body works first one side and then the other, rather than both together. These are also movements we see in many sports, for instance when reaching for a forehand at squash, or an off-drive in cricket.

In a similar way to the squatting and bending exercises, these movements target the lower body. They have a high degree of crossover with modern life and human movement, and strengthen the muscles around the buttocks and legs. They can also be equally effective as a cardiovascular exercise, particularly if done in a circuit with other exercises.

Always make sure that you maintain a good posture when lunging, ensuring that you keep your hips and shoulders level, and your knees in line with your feet.

The complex nature of these exercises challenges the core muscles, but it is the hips and legs that are required to do most of the work. Make sure the movements are controlled and pay attention to keeping good form throughout.

Basic lunge

This simple exercise is the basic starting point for the rest of the lunging movements.

- Start with your feet shoulder-width apart and the hands held at the hips.

- Keeping your trunk upright, lunge forwards, keeping your feet shoulder-width apart.

- Lower your hips towards the floor under control.

- Do not let the rear knee touch the floor.

- Return to the start position and repeat with the opposite leg.

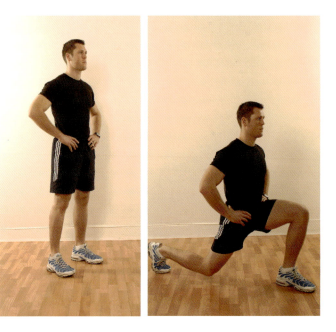

Twisting lunge

This is another variation on the basic lunge movement.

- Perform this exercise as for the basic lunge.

- Hold your arms out in front with your fingers interlocked at shoulder-height.

- As you lunge forwards, rotate your upper body towards the lead leg.

- Alternate movements on each leg.

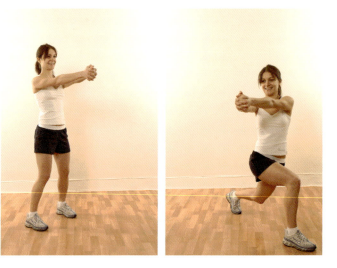

Step-ups

Not only does this exercise really strengthen the bum and thighs, it's also a great movement for getting the heart pumping and the whole body working. You can use any step you want for this; the higher the step, the greater the challenge. Be sure to place the whole foot on the step as you do the exercise.

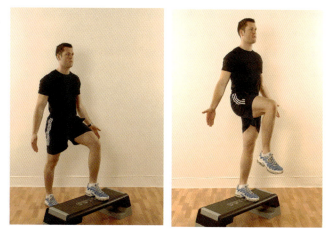

- Start with your feet shoulder-width apart and keep good posture during the movement.

- Step up with one foot, keeping your knee over your toes.

- Thrust your body upwards and into a balanced position, as shown.

- Alternate movements on each leg.

Clockface lunges

The clockface lunge is an excellent exercise for developing strength and stability in all three

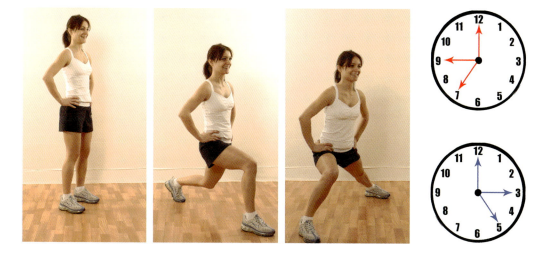

95

planes of movement. This exercise simply combines the basic lunge, shown earlier, into a sequence of movements based on an imaginary clockface drawn on the floor.

■ Start with your feet shoulder-width apart and your hands on your hips.

■ Lunge straight ahead with the left leg first (to the 12 o'clock position).

■ Return to the start position, then lunge to the side (9 o'clock).

■ Lastly, turn and lunge behind you (7 o'clock).

■ Repeat on the right side (12, 3 and 5 o'clock).

Reaching lunges

This movement is one of the most functional exercises you can do. The reaching action gives added challenge to the hips and core muscles. The movement should come mostly from your hips, not your upper back.

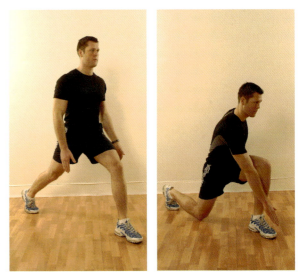

■ Face ahead with your feet around shoulder-width apart.

■ Lunge forwards, keeping your knee aligned over your toes.

■ Reach forwards with your opposite hand towards the lead ankle.

■ Repeat on the other side.

SUMMARY

These exercises in MBRT only scratch the surface of the possible types of movements that you can use to improve your strength and fitness. Often, the only limiting factor to creating exercises is your own imagination, but to help you along with adding your own variations, I have supplied a few simple suggestions below of ways to adapt and alter the exercises to suit your needs, along with some top tips to ensure you keep training safely.

- Use both bilateral and unilateral movements: Sounds complicated? It is actually very simple – bilateral simply means you are working both sides of the body at a time. Unilateral means only one side. Doing an exercise one arm or one leg at a time places a greater demand on the core of the body to keep you stabilised, and generally increases the difficulty of a movement.

- Start simple before getting complex: This old rule is very straightforward. If you haven't trained before, the easier movements are the best place to start. Learn to walk before you try to run.

- More haste, less speed: Speed is a great way to hide poor form, and although there is a place for performing exercises quickly, this shouldn't be attempted until a good base of strength has been developed. Always lift and lower under control.

- Stable to unstable: Start your movements in as stable an environment as is safe. As you progress in your skill and control, you can start to make them more challenging through use of stability challenges.

- Increase the challenge if it gets too easy: If you don't, you won't see the results.

- Maintain normal breathing through each exercise: Holding your breath can cause potentially dangerous changes in blood pressure.

- Always use a full, but pain-free, range of movement.

- Combine movements if time is short: As you get more skilled, you can start to add movements together to create your own exercises. This will not only add increased challenge to your workouts, but will also save time. Here are a few to get you started:

  - Squat to press

  - Lunge and pull

  - Step up and press.

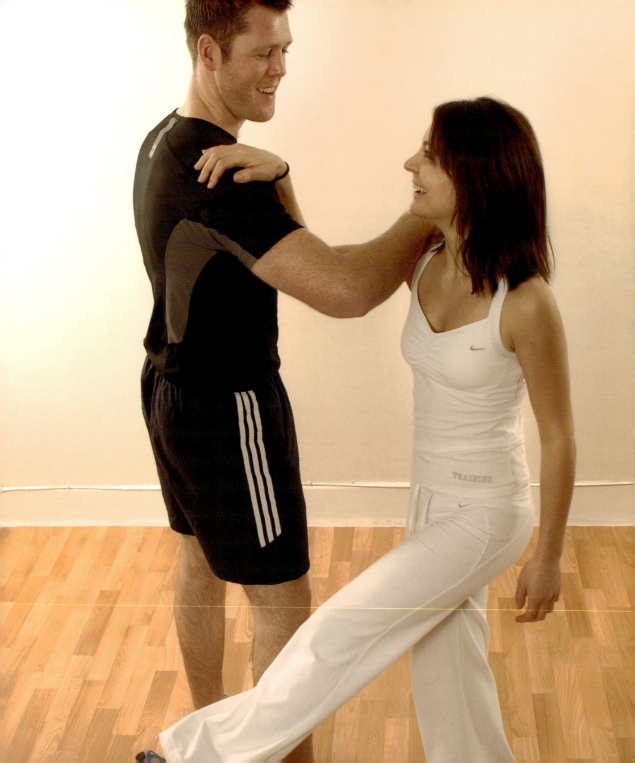

Getting the Body Ready for Action

7

The conventional approach to warming up has often been to recommend 10 minutes of light cardiovascular work, followed by a whole body stretch to 'loosen up', and then into the main workout. This somewhat dated system does not prepare our bodies for a resistance training workout, or many other activities. This chapter presents an alternative system for warming up, using functional movements that will prepare the muscles, joints, cardiovascular system and nervous system for performing at their best during the workout.

You wouldn't go for a jog before you mowed the lawn or cleaned the car, and even if you did, it wouldn't improve your performance or reduce the risk of injury. So, let's look at the reasons behind warming up and why this approach doesn't best prepare us for movement-based resistance training, core training, or balance training.

The warm-up is all about preparing the body for physical activity. Unfortunately, there is still a fair bit of misinformation and disagreement about what makes for an effective warm-up, particularly for resistance training. So, while everyone agrees that we should warm up, how we do it is a different matter.

The warm-up has a few specific purposes:

- improves movement patterns and coordination;
- increases blood flow to the muscles;
- prepares the nervous system for increased activity;
- speeds muscle contraction and relaxation;
- aids mental preparation;
- increases muscle temperature;
- improves joint mobility and movement.

A warm-up is an essential part of any workout or competition, no matter what level you are at. Although many people believe it prevents injury, it is still possible to injure yourself during a warm-up if the movement is not done correctly. So far, however, the benefits of a warm-up for performance are clearer in the research than benefits for injury prevention, and most sports and exercise scientists would agree that some form of warm-up is both advisable and beneficial for everyone before exercise.

An effective start to any training routine is to prepare the body for what lies ahead. It should contain movements that will activate our muscles ready for what is to come, and should challenge all the body's systems. So, although walking may be a good way to increase bloodflow around the body, it does not work the muscles of the hips, spine and shoulders in the way that they will be needed for exercises such as squats or press-ups. A complete warm-up will need to include activities similar to the main workout. This is the reason why athletes will prepare for their event by doing a less intense version of the real thing. An example of this is a tennis player, who will practise serving and volleying with their coach or opponent to warm up. A cyclist will prepare by cycling; it seems like common sense, right?

To prepare you for the training in this book, we are going to use active warm-up drills. By using movements similar to those in the workout ahead, but at a lower intensity, we can prepare the body for activity. The dynamic warm-up will raise the heart rate and body temperature, while also working the muscles in a way that really prepares them for the workout ahead.

Why warm up differently for cardiovascular exercise?

For cardiovascular exercise, it is particularly important that you perform a thorough warm-up using a similar (or the same) activity. As with all warm-ups, it should be both *gradual* and *progressive* to allow the body time to adapt to the change in activity levels. Suddenly beginning strenuous exercise can lead to a situation where the body is unable to keep up with the heart's need for oxygen, which can be potentially very dangerous, but which is easily avoided with a short warm-up. Begin a cardiovascular warm-up gently, and gradually increase it to the pace you are going to be training at in the workout. It is not necessary to do a full dynamic warm-up before a more gentle activity such as walking or cycling, although it certainly won't do you any harm either.

THE 10-MOVE DYNAMIC WARM-UP

The 10-move dynamic warm-up drill gets the whole body ready for activity, mobilising joints, activating muscles and preparing the mind and body for exercise. Perform this before any workout you do to help activate the muscles and nerves ready for exercise. Go through the movements continuously from start to finish, performing each 10 times, and then repeat. Gradually increase the speed and range of each exercise, starting gently and slowly, and building to a more dynamic movement.

Cats and dogs

This is a popular yoga movement and is excellent for getting the whole spine moving.

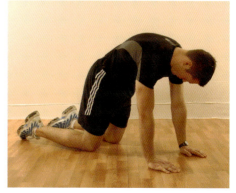

- Start on all fours with your knees and hands directly under your hips and shoulders.

- Let your chest sink to the floor and your lower back arch. Feel your tummy move towards the floor. Look up to the ceiling as you do this.

■ Then pull your tummy inwards and upwards, round your upper back, and move through a full range of motion. Let gravity take your head, and relax your neck muscles.

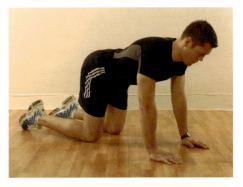

Cervical mobilisation

To further mobilise your neck, move to a standing position.

■ Look over your left shoulder, then the right. Then allow your chin to relax onto your chest.

■ Take your left ear to your left shoulder, then the right ear to the right shoulder.

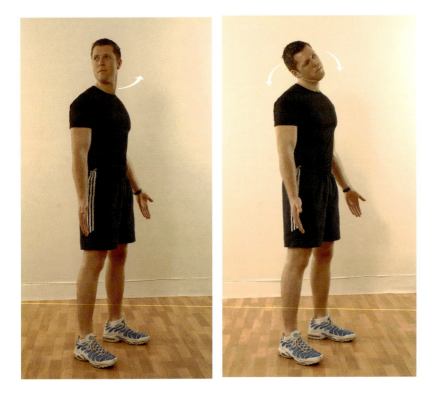

Upper body PNF (shoulder and trunk)

PNF patterns use spiral and diagonal movements to get as many muscles into the movement as possible. They also make great exercises, as well as warm-up movements.

- Start with your arms crossed over each side of your knees, palms facing backwards.

- Extend and stand up from this position. As you do this, rotate your arms as if you were drawing a sword. Feel your body opening out and, as your arms extend, turn your thumbs upwards and backwards.

- Return to the start position and repeat.

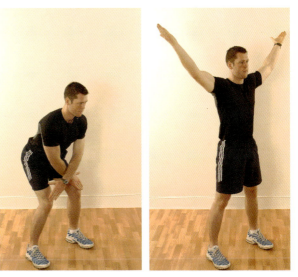

Wood chops

This movement recreates an age-old pattern and follows on perfectly from the PNF patterns.

- Interlock both hands together as if clasping an axe overhead.

- Bring both hands down and across your body as if chopping wood with an axe.

- Coordinate your breathing with each axe chop.

- Keep the movement in both directions controlled and focus on bending from the hips as opposed to the upper back.

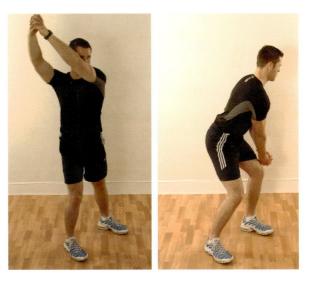

Torso twists

This classic of warm-up movements targets the muscles of the torso that control and generate rotation.

- Take your arms up to shoulder height.

- Rotate your trunk to the left and then to the right.

- Allow your hips to move; most of the rotation should come from your upper back. Do *not* force your lower back into rotation.

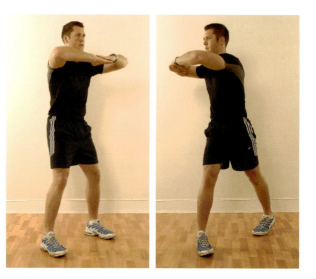

Side bends

This is another classic and effective movement.

- Place your hands by your sides, keeping good posture.

- Keeping your trunk upright, bend over to each side of the body.

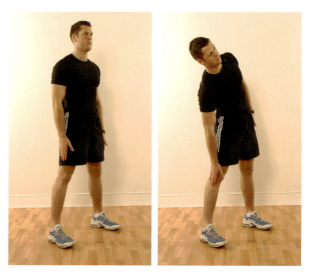

Knee raises

This movement will fire up the hips for action and also help activate the core muscles. However, take care to do the movement properly. Focus on not bending forwards in the upper back when you do it. This exercise is basically marching on the spot. Use your arms in an exaggerated marching motion to help target the shoulders as well.

- Lift your knee up until your thigh is parallel with the ground.

- Keep your torso upright.

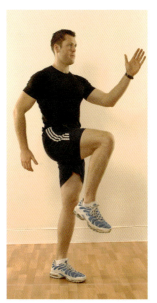

Hip swings

Find something to lean on for balance when starting out on this exercise. You can use a wall or sturdy chair for support.

- Start by taking your leg back from standing. Keep good posture when you do this and do not arch the lower back.

- Using the muscles at the front of your hip, swing your leg through and upwards. Do not force this movement.

- As your leg swings back, allow your knee to bend, bringing your heel towards your backside.

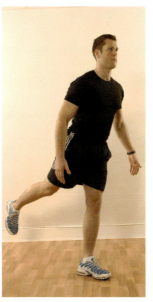

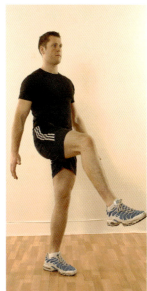

Lunge

Lunging is a really dynamic movement and a great general exercise to get the large muscles of the hip and legs moving in a functional pattern.

- Start with your feet hip-/shoulder-width apart.

- Lunge forwards, keeping your torso upright and your knee over your toes.

- Alternate legs.

See chapter 6 for a more in-depth description of the lunge.

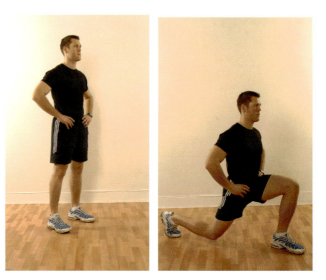

Squat and throw

The final movement of the warm-up drill is a combination of a squat exercise with a throwing movement.

- Perform the squat as outlined in chapter 6.

- During the descent, allow your arms to drop between your legs (you can do this using a medicine ball, dumbbell or similar resistance).

- As you extend back up, bring your arms overhead as if you were throwing an object behind you (if you are using a weight, don't actually throw it).

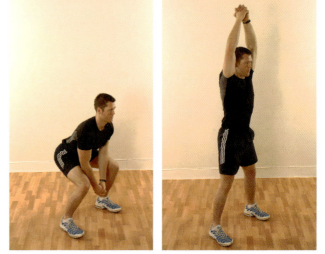

Remember, start each movement slowly, and gradually build up speed and range of motion with each repetition. Do each movement 10 times (on each side) before moving onto the next. Go through the whole drill and then repeat it. Take care to control each movement and not to bounce into any drill, as this can cause damage to muscles.

ACTIVE COOL–DOWN

The cool-down is a lot less discussed in the sports science and fitness world, yet it still serves a very important function. The cool-down is a time for reflection and recovery from the workout you have performed, and an opportunity to clear the muscles of all the by-products that our metabolisms build up during a session. It is a time to mentally and physically unwind and to enjoy the feel-good sensation that working out brings.

For that reason, the cool-down is performed on the floor. This allows quicker recovery, better return of blood to the heart, and a deeper sense of relaxation. During this routine (which you can perform as many times as needed), focus on deep rhythmic breathing and allow any remaining tension to leave the body. Perform each movement five to 10 times, stretching gently and with the minimum of effort. Combined with your essential stretches, this can make an excellent stretching session in its own right, bringing deep relaxation and a feeling of being energised; ideal after a long, hard day.

Supine lower back – lower back, hips
Do not perform this stretch if you have any disc problems with the lower back.

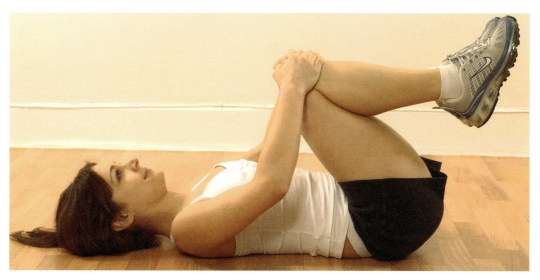

- Draw both your legs up towards your chest, taking hold of them with your arms.
- Gently pull your knees in towards your chest.
- Breathe out as you perform the movement, feeling your back relax.

Lying spinal rotation – spinal rotators/trunk

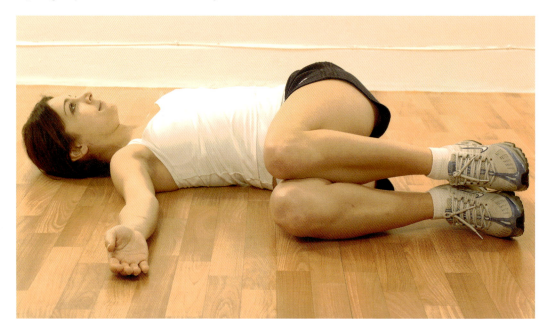

- Start with your feet flat on the floor, with knees and hips both flexed.
- Keeping your shoulders on the floor, allow your legs to slowly drop to the side.
- Breathe out as you lower.
- Return to the middle and lower to the opposite side.

Active lying hamstring – posterior thigh/hip muscles

- Take hold of one leg behind the knee and bring it in towards your chest.

- Keeping your pelvis in a neutral position, slowly extend your leg towards the ceiling until you feel the stretch in the back of your leg.

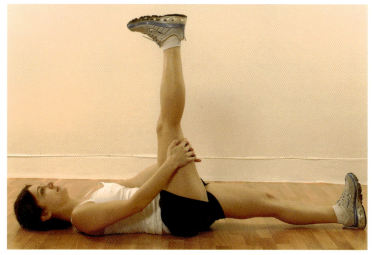

Pretzel position – hip rotators

- Start with both feet flat on the floor, with hips and knees flexed.

- Cross your right leg over your left.

- Reach around the left leg, and take a hold of it behind the knee.

- Gently lift your leg upwards and in towards your chest until you feel a stretch in your bum.

- Ease into the movement and gently repeat before changing sides.

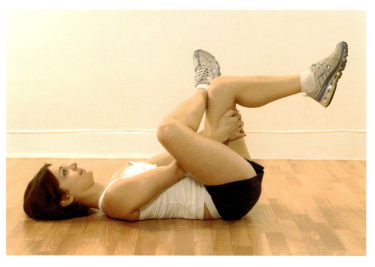

Round the clock – trunk

- Lie on your side with your knees bent and drawn towards your chest, and both hands together palm to palm.
- Using your top hand, slowly trace a line around your head, as if it were the big hand on a large clock.
- Allow your shoulders to open out and your trunk to slowly rotate over onto your back. Keep the movement slow and gentle.

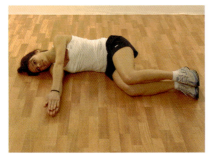

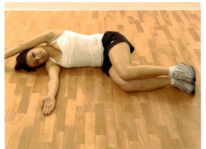

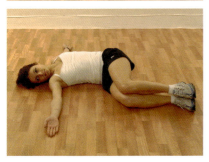

Mckenzie press-up – thoracic spine and lumbar region

Do not perform this movement if you are suffering any acute back problems.

- Start this movement on your front.
- Place your hands by your shoulders, palms on the floor.
- Take a deep breath in and, as you breathe out, slowly press with your hands and lift your body upwards.
- Keep your pelvis on the floor; do not allow your hips to lift.
- As you press up, gently ease your chest forwards.

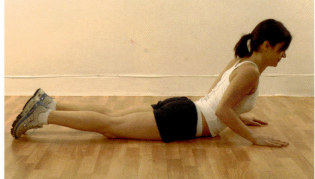

Cats and dogs – thoracic spine

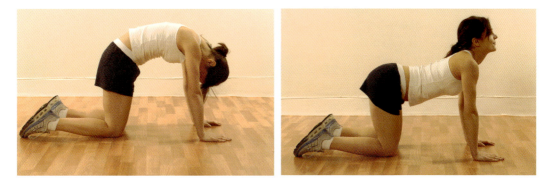

- Start on all fours with your knees and hands directly under your hips and shoulders.

- Let your chest sink to the floor and your lower back to arch. Feel your tummy move towards the floor. Look up to the ceiling as you do this.

- Then pull your tummy inwards and upwards; round your upper back and move through a full range of motion. Let gravity take your head, and relax the neck muscles.

Quadruped rocks – trunk/back

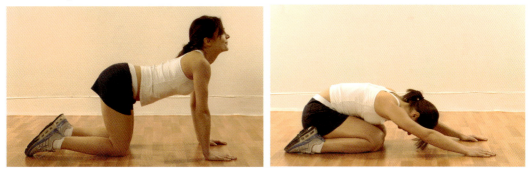

- From the same position as the previous movement, slowly allow your hips to sink backwards towards your feet.

- Allow your head to relax downwards and keep your arms out in front.

- Slowly move back to the start position and repeat.

111

Kneeling lunge – hips

- Place one leg back behind you and bring the other one to the front, in a similar position to a runner in the blocks. You may need to use a chair or something similar to aid balance when you first try this one.

- Slowly bring your trunk upright and allow your hip to sink forwards, feeling a stretch at the front of your thigh and hip.

- Once you have mastered balance, bring the arm of the side you are stretching upwards, and reach up and across your body to increase the stretch.

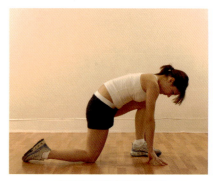

Total body PNF – total body

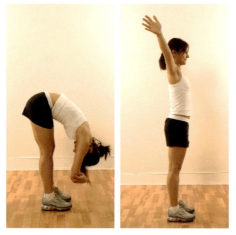

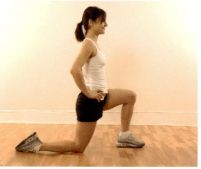

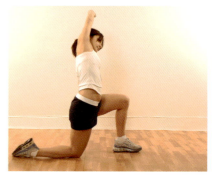

- Allow your body to hang down, keeping your arms and shoulders totally relaxed.

- Breathing deeply, slowly stand upright. Open out your arms, turning your thumbs upwards and backwards.

- Feel your chest expand and a deep stretch through your ribs and trunk.

- Repeat as many times as needed to achieve a feeling of deep relaxation.

SUMMARY

Warming up and cooling down are often the neglected parts of any exercise routine and are frequently skipped to get to the main workout or showers. Many people mentally 'switch off' during the warm-up or cool-down, but this is the best time to gain mental focus. Use my four top tips below to get more from your pre- and post-workout routines.

1 During the warm-up, focus on visualising the workout ahead. Many athletes use this time to mentally sharpen and rehearse performance. Visualise the exercises ahead and see yourself achieving each one successfully.

2 Treat each warm-up and cool-down movement as an exercise in its own right. Take time to learn them and work through them with precision and patience.

3 During the cool-down, focus on achieving a feeling of relaxation by coordinating breathing with movements. Concentrate on each movement and feel your muscles relax into each repetition. Reflect on your workout and be positive about taking a step closer to achieving your goals.

4 Consider the use of music to help; something upbeat and lively is perfect for the warm-up, while something relaxing and of a slower tempo is more suited to the cool-down.

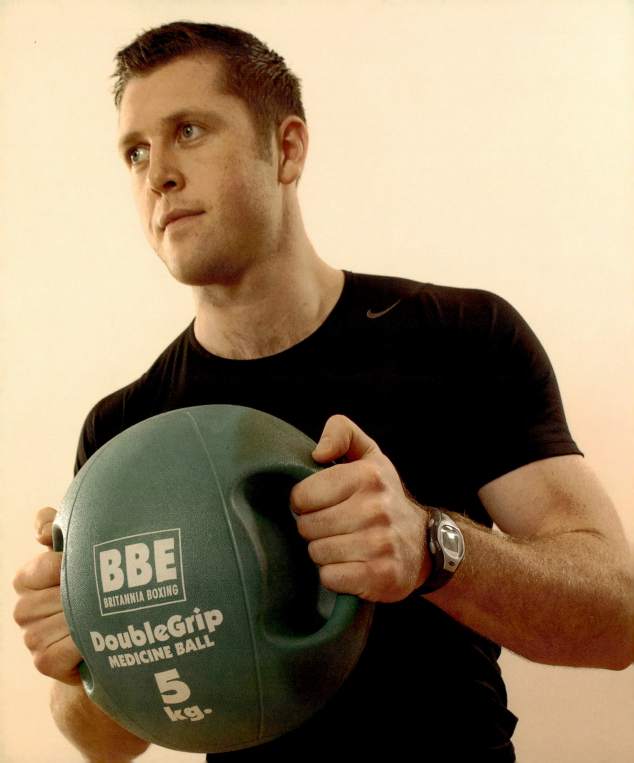

Cardiovascular Training – Developing a Healthy Heart and Lungs

8

The heart is the engine room of the body. Along with the lungs, it is responsible for the supply and extraction of everything that the body needs to work, and its function is critical to our survival. But the heart is a muscle, and like all our other muscles it is susceptible to change with age and inactivity. The ability of our heart and lungs to function effectively limits how hard we can work. Inactivity plays a large part of this, leading to loss of muscle, increase in weight, and a reduction in the ability of our bodies to effectively use energy.

As mentioned at the start of this book, these changes are reversible. With exercise training, it is possible to have a massive effect on how we age and function, allowing us to live healthy and active lives for many more years.

So, what exactly is cardiovascular training? Some might say running or cycling, but the term cardiovascular exercise could describe any activity that raises our heart rate and increases blood-flow around the body. What most of us think of as being 'cardio work' is actually *aerobic training* (with oxygen). This simply means that it is being done at a level where the body is able to use oxygen at a steady rate (hence the expression 'steady-state training') to supply energy to the muscles. Jogging and cycling are good examples of this, where we can sustain the activity as long as our energy reserves allow, provided we don't work too hard.

In contrast, *anaerobic training* (without oxygen) is done when the demand for energy is so great that we need to rely on other systems of energy delivery to keep us working. This system of energy release is very limited, and although it can supply energy fast, it also runs out quickly. Another cost of this fast delivery of energy is a build-up of substances in the muscle that can cause fatigue; slowing down or stopping what you're doing is the only way to relieve this. Weight training helps to train our system for anaerobic work, so this chapter will concentrate primarily on *aerobic* exercise. It is important to remember that both *weight training* and *aerobic training* have *positive* effects on our health.

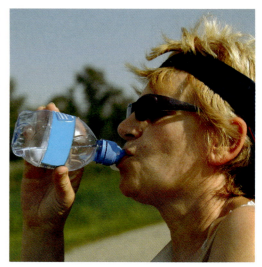

Energy systems at work

Whenever we do any exercise, we work both anaerobically and aerobically. The reason for this is that our aerobic system takes a few minutes to get going delivering energy to the body. This is why a progressive warm-up is important before running or cycling; if we start out too hard, our bodies can't keep up with demand for energy and we have to slow down or even stop to allow recovery.

All our energy systems overlap in how we use them. A simple example of this would be running to catch a bus. After a short dash from a standstill, you would find yourself breathing heavily. The reason for this is that we have been working anaerobically to supply energy for the quick sprint. Now that is over, we are breathing hard to use oxygen to replace that lost energy and clear out the effects of the hard sprint.

BENEFITS OF AEROBIC EXERCISE

This is one of the most researched areas of exercise science, and the benefits are well proven across the board. Just about everyone will benefit from increasing their activity levels, but those who are currently inactive will gain the most. In a similar way to strength training, moderate aerobic activity (doing something that makes you sweat and breathe harder) has significant effects, such as:

- making everyday tasks easier and less tiring;

- improving performance in our work, sport and recreation;

- improving the health of our heart and lungs;

- reducing the risk of death and serious illness, particularly from heart disease, various cancers, diabetes, high blood pressure, depression, osteoporosis and stroke;

- counteracting the life-shortening effects of obesity, smoking, drinking and inactivity;

- improving how we look, feel and function.

It has even been shown that regular aerobic exercise can help counteract genetics. Statistics show that losing a parent to illness before the age of 65 puts the child at a far greater risk of illness and premature death, yet regular exercise has been shown to reduce risk of this by 25 per cent. As shown in chapter 1, exercise has beneficial effects on all manner of conditions including gallstones, asthma, anxiety, insomnia, stress, hearing problems, Alzheimer's disease (by maintaining health and reducing agitation), Parkinson's disease, and in recovery and rehabilitation from many surgical procedures.

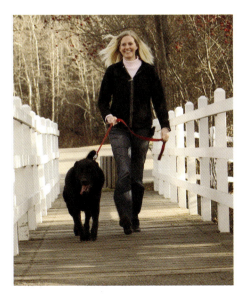

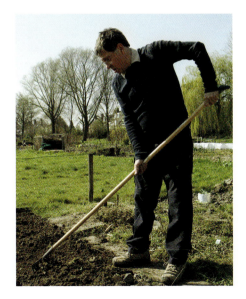

Why just doing something is better than nothing

Training for fitness is very different from training for health benefits. To improve fitness, we need to train with enough intensity to keep us improving, but to improve our health we simply need to get more active. From being inactive to doing something that involves movement, such as gardening or walking, you can considerably decrease your risk of serious illness in later life. Research has shown that regular walkers reduce their risk of a first heart attack by 73 per cent, and those who gardened regularly reduced their risk by 66 per cent compared with others who did nothing. It's not only heart attacks that activity helps to prevent, either; being active can also have a significant effect on preventing many common diseases such as diabetes and high blood pressure, and even certain types of cancers. Many of these benefits come from the type of activities that may not be 'fitness-related' but still have substantial impact on our health, and go to show that doing something is a lot better than doing nothing at all.

SO, IS AEROBIC TRAINING THE BEST WAY TO LOSE WEIGHT?

Sorry, but I'm afraid the answer to this is no. Over the last few years, a great deal of emphasis has been placed on low-level, slow, steady-state aerobic exercise for health and weight loss. Exercise programmes have been devised for people to work in their 'fat-burning zone' for optimal weight loss, and low-intensity aerobic training has become very popular for this reason.

The truth is that the 'fat-burning zone' exercise is like the Emperor's new clothes. For most of us, the idea of a magical exercise level that sheds fat with little effort simply doesn't exist, and training at low-level heart rates to try to keep yourself in your 'fat-burning zone' is unlikely to get you the results you want.

While it is true that we use fat as our main source of fuel when doing low-intensity exercise, the fact remains (*see* chapter 1) that losing excess weight is about burning calories, and if you are hardly sweating or breathing harder while exercising, then you are probably not getting through too many of those!

The common gym myth that lots of aerobic training is the best way to lose weight has led to many people (women in particular) overdosing on 'cardio machines' and avoiding weight training, often for fear of developing too much muscle.

Research has proven that for the best results in weight loss, as well as general health improvement, aerobic training is most effective when combined with resistance training. Remember, it is muscle that burns fat. So, if we can maintain or improve our muscle, we will be burning more fat, 24 hours a day. Not only that, but when we have greater variety in what we do, there's a far better chance that we'll keep doing it.

PROGRESSION

One of the first principles you learn about when studying exercise science is that of *overload*. Just as with resistance training, the cardiovascular system improves by being stimulated with an overload. It then reacts to this by becoming stronger and more efficient. To maintain these changes, we need to keep progression in our exercise.

Without progression, we stop getting results, and often lose motivation and interest. An example of this is going to a weekly exercise class such as aerobics. Many people start classes and get good results, but find that over time they stop seeing improvements in their body. It is not uncommon to find many people who have been going to the same class for months, even years, who are still overweight.

This is because one of the problems with steady-state aerobic work is that the only way to progress is to just go on longer and longer. This can lead to injuries and overtraining (where performance starts to suffer from doing too much), although more often than not, the problem is boredom and lack of motivation.

Even the most hardened of elite athletes will sometimes find it hard to find the motivation to go out and train, so it is no surprise that the thought of an hour on the treadmill at the local gym four or five times a week doesn't exactly sound either fun or exciting!

INTERVAL TRAINING – GETTING MORE BANG FOR YOUR BUCK

One of the easiest ways to add variety and progression to your aerobic training is to use a system known as *interval training*. Research has shown that as well as making huge improvements in aerobic fitness, interval training can also improve our ability to work anaerobically – something steady-state training simply doesn't do.

First developed many years ago for use by athletes, this simple technique involves a period of work followed by a period of active recovery. It is popular among many athletes for improving their ability to work at a higher level than they could sustain for the duration of their event, although the same principles have been used in rehabilitation of cancer patients, and in people with respiratory and heart problems who may find it hard to sustain a desired workrate for very long.

Interval training can be effective for everyone, and two key things dictate the challenge of the workout:

1 How hard you work during the work phase;

2 How long you allow for the recovery phase.

Let's look at a simple format – we'll call it lamppost training. This an excellent way to improve your running if you are just starting out.

Many people find it hard to sustain a steady running pace when they first start, and often tire quickly. Lampposts are regularly spaced and provide easy landmarks for this simple drill.

1 Begin with a gentle warm-up.

2 Walk briskly for the distance it takes to pass three lampposts.

3 Jog or run for the distance it takes to get past another lamppost.

4 Repeat steps 2 and 3. This is one interval.

You can repeat this as many times as you like for the workout. To add a progression, try to shorten the recovery period. For example, instead of passing three lampposts during your recovery, only pass two. This allows you to work on your running fitness without becoming too tired early in your workout.

You can also use timings as another method for this. Initially begin with a longer recovery period as above. An example of a timed interval workout is below.

■ Start with a gentle warm-up.

■ Walk at a brisk pace for two minutes.

■ Run for 30 seconds.

■ Repeat steps 2 and 3. This is one interval.

The timings and the intensity at which you work are all down to you. An experienced runner may use a short recovery period that is a similar time to the work period. For improving fitness, the key is in the intensity of the work intervals.

In contrast, someone with high blood pressure or heart disease would not work at the very high level of intensity that an athlete might, though the principle of using active recovery along with a shorter, but harder, work period would be the same. The key to the success of this format is progression; if it is too easy, either shorten the recovery time or increase the intensity of the work period. Simple and very effective, this format can be used by anyone looking to improve endurance or body composition.

Measuring intensity – how hard is hard enough?

Many different methods exist for measuring how hard you are working while exercising. These range from the scientific, such as recording a heart rate, through to the more subjective, such as grading your work level from one to 10.

Remember, the key is that you need overload to get progression, but it doesn't need to be exhausting to be effective. Moderate exercise should get you breathing hard, but *you should still be able to manage a conversation*. If you are barely breaking a sweat and it feels relatively easy, you probably need to work a bit harder. One method of measuring how hard you are working is to use your rate of perceived exertion or RPE. This system provides a more subjective way of gauging intensity, though it isn't always very accurate. People new to exercise or who are unfit will always tend to overestimate their score, while experienced athletes tend to do the opposite. A simple example of RPE is on a scale of 1–10.

1 Very gentle – no effort at all needed
2
3 Gentle – little effort but noticeable
4 Light – easily sustainable with some effort
5
6 Moderate – challenging but sustainable
7
8 Hard work – difficult to maintain
9
10 Extremely hard – maximum effort

For your cardio training to be effective, it should involve some time spent working at around level 6. Of course, one person's idea of hard work is different from another's, and no method is without drawbacks, but if you are honest with yourself you probably won't be far off the mark.

WARMING UP AND COOLING DOWN

Every cardio training workout you do should include a thorough warm-up and cool-down. Chapter 7 covers the importance and benefits of preparing the body for activity, and in particular how it is most effective to use exercises for the warm-up that help prepare the right muscles and movements for your main workout. So, if your chosen activity is running, then jogging at a lower intensity is a good way to get warmed up; similarly, if you are going out cycling, taking the first 10 minutes or so at a gentle pace is an ideal warm-up.

The warm-up is particularly important when we are giving the heart and lungs a good workout or if you suffer from a medical condition, such as high blood pressure, diabetes or asthma, as it gives the body time to adjust to the increased demand for the oxygen that it needs for exercise.

Always start all your aerobic training sessions with a thorough warm-up, starting out at around 50 per cent of your effort and progressing up to the level you plan to work at over the following five to 10 minutes.

PLANNING YOUR CARDIO TRAINING

The cardio training in this programme is simple and easy to perform, and though it may be a bit harder work than the long/slow approach, it will bring far greater benefits to your fitness, health, and weight loss goals.

To begin with, the main focus should be on simply getting moving three times a week for around 20–30 minutes at a time. If done correctly, cardio training can be an effective way to improve your fitness and health. It can also be a great way to lose body fat and improve body composition. However, aerobic exercise *alone* is not the way forward to improve your health and fitness. It doesn't address the critical importance of strength, power, flexibility, maintenance of muscle, and neural function, which are all qualities that, if compromised, will contribute to a poorer functioning of our cardiovascular system and the body as a whole.

For the best results, aerobic exercise should be combined with whole body resistance training and movement such as the programmes shown in this book.

To plan your cardio training, head to chapter 10 where we put everything together to make your workout and to get you stronger and fitter, for life!

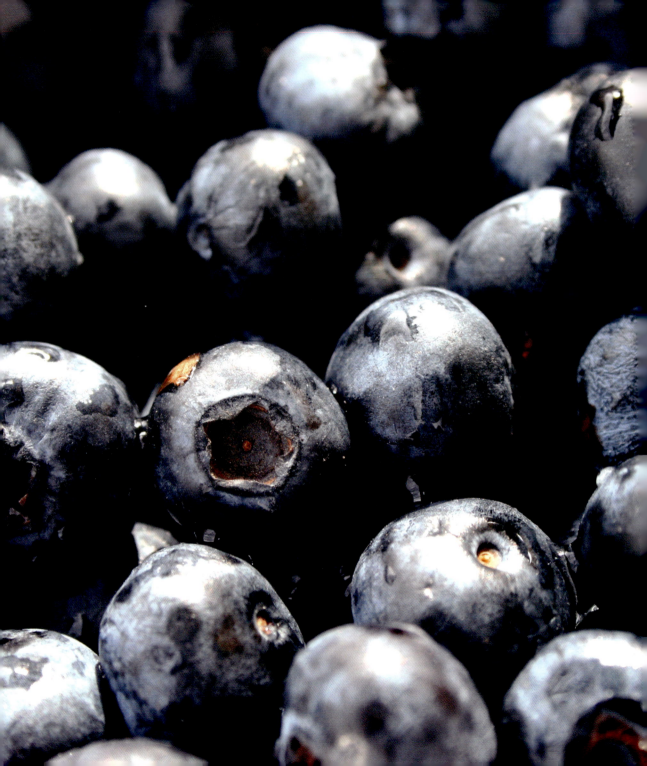

Nutrition – Supporting Your Training Through a Healthy Lifestyle

9

It seems hard to switch on the TV or pick up a paper these days without seeing something on diet and nutrition. From the latest celebrity diet to the reality TV food guru, there is no shortage of information on how to have a healthier approach to eating. There are also countless books on the subject that go into great detail on the science of how to eat more healthily. Many of these books contain a wealth of excellent information and their own ideas on the best approach to a better way of eating.

An active lifestyle gets its best results when supported with a good diet. So, I have given you my ten top tips on how to sustain a healthy and happy approach to eating. Of course, this isn't a nutrition book, so you'll have to take my word for it on the science. What I am saying is by no means complete, but this simple advice is all you need to get started on making positive changes to how you eat.

Changing diet can be difficult for some people. Often, we use excuses such as a lack of time or money for not eating well. Try to remember that your health should be your top priority, and that making a little extra time to prepare a decent meal instead of reaching for the microwave chips will make all the difference to your overall health.

These tips are in no particular order, though some are perhaps more critical to optimum health than others. Follow this advice and you will be on your way to better all-round health. Many of my clients have had great results and so will you. It is important to remember that eating well is about more than losing weight. How we eat affects our body's ability to renew, repair and prevent illness. This can change how we age, preventing wrinkles (often caused by poor hydration), reducing hair loss and improving essential fat absorption (through better protein digestion), as well as protecting our heart, liver, bones, hormones, and immune system.

1 Drink plenty of water. Most people are chronically dehydrated from simply not taking in enough water. Water serves so many fundamental roles in the body, from cell production to temperature regulation, and is essential to life. Much of the weight of the upper body is supported on discs in the lower back that are made up of 75 per cent water!

For many, the solution to thirst is to drink coffee, tea, fizzy drinks or alcohol. However, each of these actually dehydrates us further, and many contain powerful stimulants such as caffeine that can override our body's natural systems, worsening the problem. Add to that the high levels of sugar they contain and you are on an express route to problems, from tooth decay to weight gain and diabetes.

Aim to drink 2–2.5 litres of bottled water a day (generally cleaner than tap water), and always have a glass of water before eating. Although reducing caffeine can be hard initially, the negative effects of it soon exit the system to leave you feeling healthier and happier. A simple test for your hydration is to check your urine colour. If you are well-hydrated, your urine should be pale or clear in colour. If it is a dark yellow, you are dehydrated and need to drink more. (If you are taking B vitamins or a multivitamin, this can change the colour of your urine to a bright yellow.)

2 Get enough sleep. Allowing the body time to recover is one of the most important parts of a healthy lifestyle, and getting enough sleep is central to that. Although this may not be about diet, what you eat can also affect how you sleep, and it is a good idea to avoid eating before you go to bed, particularly sugary foods. Good-quality sleep is essential for us to feel energised and recovered. Without it, the adrenal hormones (in particular, cortisol) do not run their natural cycle and stay chronically elevated. This vicious circle can lead to an increased risk of weight gain, diabetes and many other health problems, as well as leaving us feeling irritable, bad-tempered, and unable to concentrate.

To get your sleep patterns back on track, establish a bedtime and a wake-up time routine. Stick to these and within a week your body will have adjusted to them, even though you may find it hard to get used to at first. You should aim for eight clear hours of sleep. It is also a good idea that before bedtime you avoid things that stimulate the mind, and try to do things that aid relaxation and rest. This could be listening to relaxing music, reading a light and easy-to-put-down book, or drinking some herbal tea.

In the evening, avoid foods that contain *tyramine*, as this increases the release of stimulants in the body that will prevent you from sleeping; caffeine, alcohol, sugar, tobacco, chocolate, wine, bacon, ham, sausage, potatoes, spinach and tomatoes all contain tyramine.

To help sleep, try to include foods that contain *tryptophan* in your evening meals; these are necessary for the release of *serotonin*, a hormone that initiates sleep. These foods include fish, chicken, turkey, bananas, figs, dates, yoghurt, tuna, eggs, soya beans, tofu, nuts, cottage cheese, avocadoes and whole grain crackers.

3 Eat enough protein. Protein is one of the main nutrients in our diet and we need it in fairly large amounts when we are training. Resistance training stimulates a breakdown in muscle proteins, so it is essential to have enough in the body to help repair and rebuild muscles. This has been shown to be particularly important in older adults, particularly after working out, for the growth of new muscle. There are varying recommendations for optimal protein intake; often people trying to gain weight will greatly increase protein to help with muscle growth. However, high protein intake is not advisable for all, as it can overwork the kidneys and upset the acid/alkaline balance in the body. This can cause a loss of minerals in the body that, in turn, can lead to osteoporosis, as *calcium* is taken from the bone to neutralise the acidity.

The best sources of protein include fish, meat, beans, lentils, eggs and soya. Many meat sources can be high in the harmful types of fat, so try not to rely on these for your protein intake. Vegetables such as broccoli, runner beans, peas and legumes contain good protein (especially when combined with whole grains), as well as being an excellent source of energy and vitamins.

4 Eat regularly. Going for many hours without eating is a sure way to find yourself reaching for that convenience food when you get the chance. Not only that, but it will lead to your metabolism slowing down as your body tries to conserve valuable energy stores. Going too long without something to eat will cause fatigue, tiredness, lethargy, and low levels of blood sugar. Many people don't eat enough throughout the day and end up having a large meal in the evening. By this time the body is so desperate for food that it will store all this energy, leaving you tired on the sofa as your body has to work to digest it all. Our preservation mode also kicks in, and any food taken after a long day without eating will be stored as fat, instead of being used for energy.

By eating small meals regularly, we can create a healthy balance in blood sugar levels, maintain energy and avoid the need for a large evening meal. Try to eat five or six times a day, and make lunch your biggest meal of the day. Remember, graze – don't gorge!

5 Be sugar-aware. Sugar is probably the biggest enemy to a healthy diet, and these days it is added to just about everything that comes packaged, tinned or boxed. When refined sugar comes in a form that is quickly absorbed into the body (white bread, white pasta, orange squash), it causes a release of *insulin* into the body. This hormone promotes the storage of sugar as fat and, over time, as fat levels increase and our sensitivity to insulin decreases, it can lead to the development of diabetes. This used to be known as adult-onset diabetes due to it affecting us in later life, but excessive sugar levels in processed foods, fizzy drinks, and junk food have now led to it being seen in teenagers. Not only this, but sugar negatively affects energy levels, and can contribute to certain types of cancer, heart disease and other illnesses, even behavioural problems!

To avoid becoming a victim of excess sugar, avoid processed foods (such as ready meals), cereals (almost all of the common breakfast cereals have added sugar), processed fruit juices, flavoured water and fizzy drinks, and refined foods. These foods contain high amounts of sugar but none of the other nutrients that you need to digest it. This also includes alcoholic drinks, which are full of calories and devoid of nutrients. Even worse, alcohol requires many essential B vitamins to metabolise, it damages the gut and liver, and blocks the absorption of many beneficial vitamins and minerals. Make a start today by cutting it from your diet. Aside from the obvious sugars we know, beware of *hidden* sugars under other names such as corn syrup, fructose, lactose, malted barley, fruit juice concentrate, and raisin syrup; if anything ends in either *syrup* or '*ose*' then it is made purely from sugar.

If you long for that sweet taste, try a few blueberries, dried apricots or a freshly prepared juice. A juicer can cost as little as £20 and there are numerous recipes around to help ease the sweetest tooth. Although fruit contains more goodness, don't go overboard with it, it's still sugar and many people find fructose (fruit sugar) difficult to digest. If you suffer from irritable bowel syndrome (IBS), then avoid citrus fruits in particular.

6 Eat the right fats. A common approach to trying to lose weight is the eradication of all the fat from your diet in favour of 'low fat' alternatives. However, not only does this approach make eating very difficult, it also ignores the fact that the body actually *needs* some fat to function properly. Our metabolism (including how we actually convert nutrients into energy) is reliant on essential fatty acids for it to function at all, and the body cannot

produce new cells without it. Most low-fat food makes up for the lack in fat with a very high sugar content, leaving you feeling empty and still hungry after you have eaten.

To get the right type of fat in your diet, avoid *saturated fats* such as those found in margarine, cheese, biscuits, crisps and fried food. Saturated fat is the fast way to gain weight and puts you at greater risk of heart disease. Instead, eat oily fish (salmon, mackerel, tuna) twice a week, unsalted nuts and seeds (keep it to a handful daily as these are very high in calories), and use extra virgin olive oil on your salads (but don't cook with it, as heating it up destroys all the goodness in it). These oils contain the essential *Omega 3 and 6* that we need to make new cells and enzymes that we need to keep joints and organs (even our brain!) healthy. Stay clear of anything containing *hydrogenated vegetable oil*, where an unnatural process is used to mass produce hard fats from liquids. This is bad for the body, as it simply cannot deal with them effectively.

7 Always eat breakfast. I have worked with many clients whose day starts off badly with either a poor breakfast, or worse, no breakfast at all. If you don't start the day on the right footing, it is always going to be a case of playing catch-up with the body for the next 24 hours. Many of the same people who neglect a proper breakfast are the same ones reliant on stimulants such as caffeine to get them through the morning.

Breakfast should be a complete meal; eat too little and you risk reaching for that sugary snack or coffee to perk you up an hour or two later. Your first meal of the day should also contain some source of protein, which helps to set the body up to regulate its blood sugar levels throughout the day. Try including such things as natural yoghurt, seeds, nuts, eggs, soya, sardines, kippers, or even chicken!

8 Get at least five a day. You may have noticed that some supermarket chains are now very gently promoting the five-a-day approach to eating fruit and vegetables. Eating your 'greens' is absolutely essential for optimum health, as they are rich in nutrients, vitamins and minerals that the body needs to function at its best. Not only that, but nobody ever got fat from eating too many vegetables, so they are excellent if you are trying to lose weight. It's not just green vegetables that are important; each colour has its own different qualities. As well as valuable vitamins, these also contain *antioxidants* that protect our bodies from damage caused from harmful chemical reactions in the body. These reactions are made worse by the chemicals, additives and pollution around us.

Fruit and vegetables are also a great source of *fibre* in the diet. Fibre is perhaps the most underrated part of people's diets in terms of the health benefits it can bring.

Low-fibre diets are associated with an increased risk of heart disease and certain cancers. Fibre is nature's great cleanser, and on its way through the body it picks up many harmful substances, and helps us to remove them regularly and easily.

If a meal lacks colour and everything on your plate is white, then it is likely that there are not enough vegetables in your diet. Try to make food as colourful as possible by adding veg to every meal. It needn't be soggy Brussels sprouts either; there are many exciting, tasty and healthy fruits and vegetables you can add to your diet for variety and enjoyment.

9 Supplement where needed. There is often a deep-rooted distrust of taking supplements as part of your diet. For many of us, these concerns are unfounded, as certain supplements can improve health, boost the immune system, reduce the impact of stress and promote the absorption and digestion of many other foods.

The quality of your supplements is important though. Many high street multivitamins, for example, are 'fast food' supplements, low on quality and produced with the cheapest available ingredients.

Supplementing can help many people with food intolerances or dietary problems, but can also be very useful to those with a healthy lifestyle. Although a full and healthy diet *should* contain enough vitamins and minerals, mass farming and low quality soils have led to our fruit and vegetables having lower levels of nutrients. This is one of the reasons that organic produce is preferable.

Before adding supplements to your diet, I recommend that you check with your doctor or see a nutritionist, as some types of supplement can be harmful to people such as pregnant women, those on medication and anyone with a specific disease or condition.

Generally, you can support your diet with a good multivitamin, extra vitamin C and a fish oil capsule. For those wanting to support bone growth, or those with insomnia, muscle cramps, stress and fatigue, you can consider the use of calcium and *magnesium*.

10 Forget dieting. The word diet actually means 'way of life', yet it seems to have become distorted over the past years to mean something else entirely. There are all kinds of diets out there, from Atkins to cabbage soup, but who wants to eat that for the rest of their life? Dieting is destined to fail long-term, and the proof is in speaking to anyone who has ever been on one. In the short-term, it leads to stress and anxiety, affecting how you feel, both inside mind and body, normally for the worse. Very few people manage to sustain healthy weight loss simply through restricting calories. This kind of social obsession leads to eating disorders, illness, depression, rapid weight loss and gain (yo-yo dieting), loss of muscle mass, a drop in metabolic rate (leading to a lower overall daily use of calories, which contributes about 75 per cent of your daily energy use), and overall poor health. Stop thinking quick-fix and start thinking about changing how you eat for good. That way, you'll have the kind of body and health you will be really happy with.

Changing how you approach your eating habits can be challenging for many people. It means taking a little more time over what and how you eat, right through from being a bit more selective in your shopping to actually spending a little longer preparing, eating and digesting your food.

To make the change easier and more focused, pick one particular tip at a time and work on making that your main nutritional focus. Once you have mastered it, take another one and go from there. As most people are chronically dehydrated when they start training, I always advise tip 1 – to drink more water – as the best place to start. Many people notice the difference from that straight away.

You could also consider visiting a nutritional therapist. Far from just giving you meal ideas, a nutritional therapist can check for food intolerances, deficiencies and hormonal imbalances, and advise you accordingly on the best foods to eat for your body.

The reality for many people is that they can make significant changes to their health by simply reducing their sugar intake, increasing their vegetable and fibre intake, and avoiding negative factors like alcohol, smoking, and fried foods. By cutting out the junk and sticking to a balanced and (where possible) organic diet, you will notice the improvements almost immediately.

Although eating organically has been expensive in the past, most leading supermarkets now carry extensive ranges of organic foods and it is no longer as pricey as it used to be.

Remember, this book is primarily about getting stronger and fitter, so the tips given here are by no means the whole story on healthy eating. They are intended to get you started in the right direction and to make some positive changes to your diet.

Making these changes can be tough at first, and is often not without setbacks or failures. Dieting equals stress; often, the focusing on where you want to be can lead to severe anxiety about weight and body image in the present. Instead, enjoy being yourself and take responsibility for your life and make the most of it. Keep a positive image of yourself and enjoy the achievements that you reach by improving your health, fitness and well-being.

Do all this, and the rest will follow.

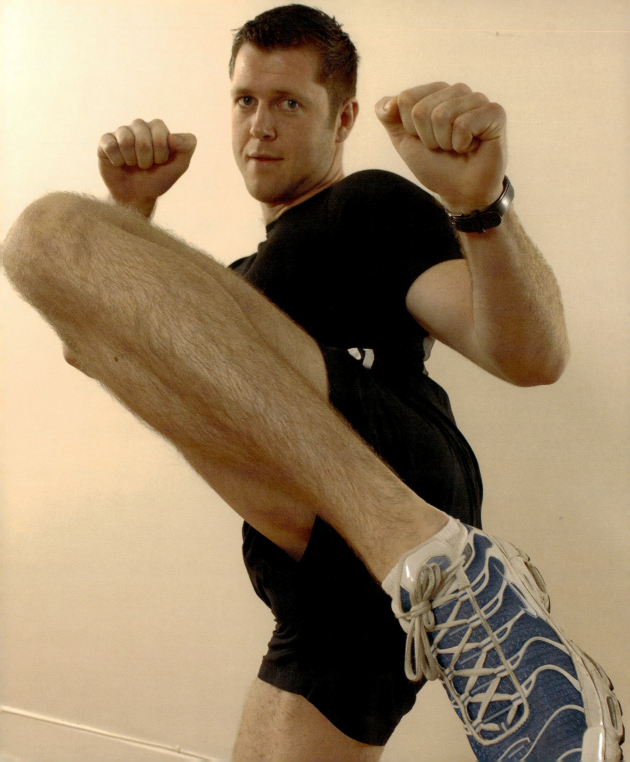

Creating Your Programme – Success by Design

10

Programme design is the bread and butter of any personal trainer, and a good understanding of it is crucial to the overall success of the workout. All the motivation, focus and energy of training can be made or broken through how the programme is put together.

In this section, we will briefly look at the essential ingredients of any training programme and how we can simply apply them to design our own unique exercise programme.

Whether you are a runner, bodybuilder, tennis player or just training to lose weight, the prerequisites are all the same for developing strength and fitness. If you have tried working out before, or are currently training and finding that the results are not coming, then the chances are that it is down to one of the following four areas.

1 Individual: Each programme needs to be individual, designed for the needs of that one person – in this case, you! There is no single ideal programme for everyone, just as there is no one size of shoe for every foot.

2 Overload: A workout provides a stimulus for the body to adapt to. If that stimulus is not enough, the body won't change and you won't get results. This becomes more important after the first six weeks of training, when most of the change comes from our body learning to exercise.

3 Progression: Without progression, the changes stop. Simply put, if you change nothing, then nothing changes. To keep your workouts fun, interesting and effective, they should change regularly.

4 Recovery: The importance of recovery and restoration is often overlooked in the fitness world where much of the discussion centres on the training itself. Recovery is the time when our body responds to the workout by building new muscle and improving systems, so it is crucial that you allow time for this to happen. How much is needed will vary from person to person, and needs to be properly supported by your diet and lifestyle.

How often should I train?

I'd recommend trying to do your programme three times a week. Remember, simply doing something is better than nothing, but you will see better results if you are able to do *something* regularly. Allow yourself time to recover after each workout (at least 24 hours). If time is short, assign priority to your essential stretches, core and balance work. *You should try and do something active most days of the week, whether it is simply taking a walk or doing some gardening.*

CREATING YOUR PROGRAMME

Creating your own programme is simple. Each programme will be arranged around the same format, although *you* pick the various stretches and exercises. Every workout you do on this programme will follow the same, easy-to-remember routine.

Step 1. Select your essential stretches based on your self-test results. These will be done first in the workout.

Step 2. The dynamic warm-up is the same for each workout. See chapter 7.

Step 3. Choose the required core exercises, based on your self-test results from chapter 2. If you have no specifics from the self-tests, simply select your own choice based on the level of difficulty you would like.

Step 4. Choose the required balance exercises.

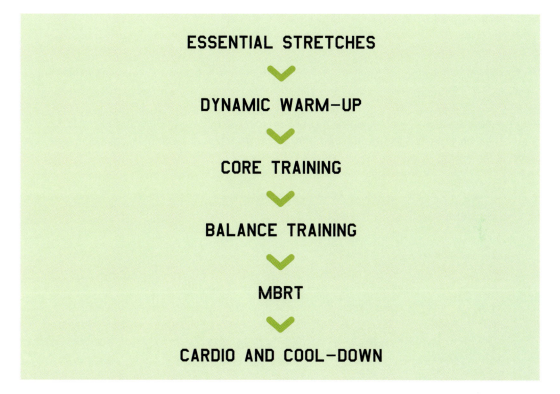

ESSENTIAL STRETCHES

DYNAMIC WARM–UP

CORE TRAINING

BALANCE TRAINING

MBRT

CARDIO AND COOL–DOWN

Step 5. Select the MBRT exercises from the options given in chapter 6, using the appropriate section for each movement pattern.

Step 6. Active cool-down is the same for each workout.

Step 7. Incorporate your cardio work.

Step 8. Start exercising and getting stronger and fitter for life!

Exercises in each phase are arranged using a simple alphabetical sequence. So, exercise A is done first, followed by B, C and so on. In phase 2 and 3 where exercises are done in combination, a number next to the letter indicates this.

To see how this works in practice, let's look at a simple example.

A1 Prisoner squats
A2 Press-up

B1 Clockface lunge
B2 Bent-over row

In this simple sequence, you would do a set of exercise A1 followed by a set of exercise A2. This would then be repeated for the desired amount of sets before beginning the combination of exercise B1 and B2.

Getting the numbers right

The number of repetitions you do for each exercise is probably the most important programme variable there is. Everyone has different fitness levels, so while one fixed range may work for some people, for others it will either be too hard or too simple.

Each exercise (with the exception of some of the core exercises) will be done with a range of between 12–16 repetitions. If you find 12 too challenging, select an easier exercise (or an easier version); conversely, if you are able to do more than 16, select either a harder level exercise or variation.

Certain core exercises are held for a period of time instead of repetitions; check each exercise for this in chapter 3.

Remember: once you can complete an exercise you have chosen for more than 16 repetitions (or recommended time), it is time to change to a harder alternative. This ensures that you progress and get better results from your training.

PHASE 1 – GETTING STARTED

When we first start to exercise, many changes are set in motion by the body. One of the first areas to improve is the body's ability to control the right muscles for a certain movement. Actual physical changes happen a lot more slowly than changes to our nervous system, which learns quickly.

The first phase is characterised by doing two sets of each exercise before moving onto the next one. The focus should be on developing a good base of movement and an improved awareness of the body before attempting more challenging combinations of exercise, such as in phase 2 and 3.

In the example shown, you can see that the only sections you have to fill in are the exercises, as the others are already complete. You would perform two sets of exercise A1 – resting for 60 seconds between each set – before moving onto exercise B1.

Cardiovascular work does not need to be done on the same day. If you are going to do your cardio work separately, go straight to the active cool-down after the resistance training. If you can, try to vary your activities, so if you walk one day, try to cycle the next.

Remember also to perform your essential stretches, dynamic warm-up and active cool-down when doing your cardiovascular work if you do perform it on a different day.

* **When putting in essential strengthening exercises, they are the priority and should always be done first.**

So, lets take a look at how a typical programme for phase 1 might look.

Section	Exercise/Stretch	Sets	Reps	Rest
Essential Stretches		3	30secs each	
Active Warm-Up				
Core or Essential A1		2	12–16	60secs then repeat
Core or Essential B1		2	12–16	60secs then repeat
Balance C1		2	12–16	60secs then repeat
Squat/Bend D1		2	12–16	60secs then repeat
Pull E1		2	12–16	60secs then repeat
Lunge/Step F1		2	12–16	60secs then repeat
CARDIO	Walking/Cycling /Swimming	2–3	10–15mins	
Active Cool-down				

PHASE 2 – STEP IT UP WITH SUPERSETS

Phase 2 builds on the work we did in phase 1 developing stability, awareness and confidence with exercising. It introduces a concept known as a 'superset'. This technique has been used successfully in exercise for years, and allows you to combine two exercises that challenge different movements. As the muscles involved are different, the performance of one exercise should not affect the other. However, this does allow us to improve fitness, cardiovascular health, coordination and endurance by reducing the amount of rest between exercises, keeping us moving for more of the workout.

Cardiovascular work in this phase introduces the *interval training* format (*see* chapter 8). This can be done either at the end of a workout or on a different day. Always remember to perform your essential stretches, dynamic warm-up and active cool-down when doing your cardiovascular work, if you are doing it separately.

Section	Exercise/Stretch	Sets	Reps	Rest
Essential Stretches		3	30secs each	
Active Warm-Up				
Core A1		2–3	12–16	None – Move to A2
Balance A2		2–3	12–16	90secs then back to A1
Squat/Bend B1		2–3	12–16	None
Pull B2		2–3	12–16	90secs then back to B1
Lunge/Step C1		2–3	12–16	None
Push C2		2–3	12–16	90secs then back to C1
CARDIO	Interval training Any activity	1	20mins	
Active Cool-down				

PHASE 3 – GET MOVING WITH CIRCUITS

The third phase of training also forms the platform for designing your continuing training programme. By this point, you should be feeling confident performing many different exercises and movements, and hopefully you are starting to feel the benefits of all the hard work you are putting in.

The third phase introduces what is known as *vertical loading* to our training – better known in the fitness world as *circuit training* – which is a fantastic way to build strength, fitness, endurance, and to improve your overall health. It combines three or more exercises done consecutively with very little rest, keeping the pulse elevated, and really challenging the heart and lungs to keep the muscles supplied with the oxygen they need to function.

Circuit training can improve both your *anaerobic* and your *aerobic* fitness as discussed in chapter 8. In this phase, you first perform a *core* and then a *balance* exercise, before performing four MBRT movements consecutively.

Cardiovascular exercise in this phase is varied, with the use of two interval-training sessions. Design these yourself based on your own fitness ability. It is important for the cardiovascular training to be varied to keep the results coming, and to prevent it from becoming boring.

Section	Exercise/Stretch	Sets	Reps	Rest
Essential Stretches		3	30secs each	
Active Warm-Up				
Core A1		2–3	12–16	30secs then onto A2
Balance A2		2–3	12–16	30secs then onto A3
Squat/Bend A3		2–3	12–16	30secs then onto A4
Lunge/Step A4		2–3	12–16	30secs then onto A5
Pull A5		2–3	12–16	30secs then onto A6
Push A6		2–3	12–16	120secs then back to A1
CARDIO	Interval training	1	30mins	
Active Cool-down				

MOVING BEYOND PHASE 3

Your training should not finish at the end of phase 3. Exercise is a lifestyle choice; if you stop exercising, you'll stop getting all those great benefits that by now you are enjoying.

You can use the programme format from phase 3 to keep your training routine up. Simply change the exercises every four to six weeks using other exercises in the book. Adding any kind of variety to your workout will be good for you. Changes in training lead to changes in the body, so to keep things going in the right direction you can, for example, try doing the exercises in the reverse order.

Cardiovascular exercise can be harder to vary, but this is important, so try to use several different methods of exercise, from swimming to running. Also, you can vary when you do it; whether you do it at the end of a workout or on a different day will make a difference.

Finally, every once in a while, take a week off. Time away from an exercise routine is important; it allows you to recharge the batteries and for your body to catch up with all the stresses you have been placing on it. Too many people have an unhealthy addiction to exercise, and though you might find it hard to imagine right now, this can lead to overtraining and exhaustion that takes a long time to recover from.

For more tips on how to vary your exercises, see chapter 6 on MBRT, and remember, each exercise in the core training section comes with a harder and easier version for you to use.

How long should I leave between workouts?

Workouts using mainly bodyweight, such as these, generally take less time to recover from. However, recovery is very important, as it is during this time that your body adapts to the stimulus of the workout.

For best results, I recommend leaving a day between each workout before repeating it. This does not mean do nothing, though! You should still include activity on these days such as walking, cycling, swimming, or even dancing!

EXERCISE QUICK REFERENCE CHART

Movement Type	Exercises	
Core	Abdominal Activation	57–8
	Leg Lock Floor Bridge	58–9
	Lower Abs Blaster	59–60
	Opposite Arm and Leg Raise	60–1
	Plank	62–3
	Prone Cobra	63–4
	Russian Twists	64–5
Balance	Single Leg Balance	73
	Clockface Reaches	74–5
	Touchdowns	75–6
	Lunge to Knee Raise	76–7
	Hop, Stop and Go	77
Squat/Bend	Basic Squat	82–3
	Split Stance Squat	83
	Overhead Squat	84
	Bulgarian Squat	84–5
	Single Leg Squat	85
Push	Wall Push-Up	86–7
	Fitball Press-Up	87
	Press-Up	87–8
	Overhead Press – Seated	88–9
	Dips	89
	Single-Arm Overhead Press	89–90
Pull	High Pulls	90
	Bent-Over Pulls	91
	Pullovers	91–2
	Archer's Pull	92
	Uppercuts	93
Lunge/Step	Basic Lunge	94
	Twisting Lunge	94
	Step-Ups	95
	Clockface Lunge	95–6
	Reaching Lunges	96

APPENDIX

Test 1	Belt Line	A	B	C
Test 2	Wall Angels	A	B	
Test 3	Forward Bending	A	B	
Test 4	Single Leg Balance	A	B	C
Test 5	Cervical Mobility	A	B	
Test 6	Chest and Shoulders	A	B	
Test 7	Hamstrings	A	B	C
Test 8	Thomas Test	A	B	
Test 9	Core Coordination	A	B	C
Test 10	Cardiovascular Health	A	B	C
	Waist/Hip Ratio (men under 60)	up to 0.9	over 0.9	
	Waist/Hip Ratio (men over 60)	up to 1.0	over 1.0	
Test 11	Waist/Hip Ratio (women under 60)	up to 0.8	over 0.8	
	Waist/Hip Ratio (women over 60)	up to 0.9	over 0.9	

Copy this chart and mark off each test from chapter 2 as you perform it. Yellow boxes indicate where there is still some room for improvement, and how you can improve by using the right exercises in your programme; green boxes show where you are performing well. Complete all the tests regularly to see if the yellows you have marked turn green – and ensure the greens you have marked before have stayed green!

BIBLIOGRAPHY AND REFERENCES

American College of Sports Medicine (1997) *Exercise Management for Persons with Chronic Disease and Disabilities*. Human Kinetics, Champaign IL, USA.

Babayak M et al (2000) Exercise treatment for major depression: Maintenance of therapeutic benefit at 10 months. *Journal of American Psychosomatic Society*. 62:633-638.

Baechle T R, Earle R (2000) *Essentials of Strength Training and Conditioning, 2nd edition*, Human Kinetics, Champaign IL.

Bahram J, *Evaluation and Retraining of the intrinsic foot muscles for pain syndromes related to abnormal control of pronation*. Advanced Physical Therapy Education Institute.

Barnett F, Gilleard W (2005) The use of lumbar spinal stabilisation techniques during the performance of abdominal strengthening exercise variations. *Journal of Sports Medicine and Physical Fitness* 45(1):38-43.

Batmanghelidj F (2000) *Your Body's Many Cries For Water*, The Tagman Press, Norwich U.K.

Berrben G (2001) The Physiology of Ageing, *ACSM Current Comments*.

Blumenthal et al (1999) Effects of exercise training on older patients with major depression. *Archives of Internal Medicine* 159(19): 2349-2356.

Braun et al (2005) Acute EPOC response in women to circuit training and treadmill exercise of matched oxygen consumption. *European Journal of Applied Physiology* 94(5-6):500-4.

Brown AB, McCartney N, Sale DG (1990) Positive adaptations to weight-lifting training in the elderly. *Journal of Applied Physiology* 69:1725-1733.

Chek P (1999) The Inner Unit: A new frontier in abdominal training. *New Studies in Athletics*.

Chek P (2004) *How to Eat, Move, and be Healthy*. C.H.E.K Institute, San Diego CA, USA.

Cook G (2003) *Athletic Body In Balance*, Human Kinetics, Champaign IL.

Delorme T L, Watkins A L (1948) Techniques of progressive resistive exercise. *Archive of Physical Medicine* 29:263.

Dunstan DW et al (2002) High-Intensity resistance training improves glycaemic control in older patients with type 2 diabetes. *Journal of Diabetes Care* 25:1729-1736.

Ebben W P, Jensen R L (1998) Strength training for women: debunking myths that block opportunity. *The Physician and Sports Medicine* 26(5).

Erasmus U (2002) *Fats that heal, Fats that kill*, Alive Books, Burnaby BC, Canada.

Escamilla R F (2000) Knee biomechanics of the dynamic squat exercise. *Medicine and Science in Sports and Exercise* 33(1) 127-141.

Evans WJ (1997) Functional and metabolic consequences of sarcopenia. *Journal of Nutrition* 127(5):998S-1003S.

Evans WJ, Campbell WW (1993) Sarcopenia and age-related changes in body composition and functional capacity, *Journal of Nutrition* 123(2 supp):465-8.

Feigenbaum MS, Pollock MS (1999) Prescription of resistance training for health and disease. *Medicine and Science in Sports and Exercise* 31(1):38-45.

Faigenbaum A (2000) Age and Sex Related Differences and Their Implications for Resistance Exercise in Baechle T R, Earle R W (2000) *Essentials of Strength Training and Conditioning*, Human Kinetics, Champaign IL.

Fiatarone MA, Marks EC, Ryan ND, Meredith CN, Lipsitz LA, Evans WJ (1990) High-intensity strength training in nonagenarians. Effects on skeletal muscle. *Journal of American Medical Association* 263(22):3029-34.

Flanagan S, Salem G J, Wang M, Sanker S E, Greendale G A (2003) Squatting exercises in older adults: kinematic and kinetic comparisons. *Medicine and Science in Sports and Exercise* 35(4): 635-643.

Fleck S J, Kraemer W J (2004) *Designing Resistance Training Programmes*, 3rd Edition. Human Kinetics, Champaign IL.

Fredericson M, Moore T (2005) Core stabilisation training for middle and long-distance runners. *New Studies in Athletics* 20(1):25-37.

Galvao DA, Taaffe DR (2005) Resistance exercise dosage in older adults: single versus multiset effects on physical performance and body composition, *Journal of American Geriatric Society* 53(12):2090-7.

Glenville M (2006) *Fat Around The Middle*, Kyle Cathie Ltd, London U.K.

Gunter et al (2000) Functional mobility discriminates non-fallers from one-time and frequent fallers. *Journal of Gerontology* 55:M672-M676.

Hall C, Brody L T (2005) *Therapeutic Exercise: Moving Toward Function*. Baltimore MA: Lippincott Williams & Wilkins.

Heitkamp et al (2001) Gain in strength and muscular balance after balance training. *International Journal of Sports Medicine* 22:285-290.

Henwood TR, Taaffe DR (2006) Short-term resistance training and the older adult: the effect of varied programmes for the enhancement of muscle strength and functional performance. *Clinical Physiology and Functional Imaging*. 26(5): 305-13.

Hertol (2000) Functional instability following lateral ankle sprain. *Journal of Sports Medicine* 29(5):361-371.

Honkola A, Forsen T, Eriksson J (1997) Resistance training improves the metabolic profile in individuals with type 2 diabetes. *Acta Diabetologica* 34(4):245-248.

Hu M H, Woollacott M H (1994) Multisensory training of standing balance in older adults: Postural stability and one-leg stance balance. *Journal of Gerontology* 49(2):52-61.

James M, Jongeward D (1996) *Born to Win*, Da Capo Press, Cambridge MA, USA.

Judge J O (2003) Balance training to maintain mobility and prevent disability. *American Journal of Preventative Medicine* 25(3 Suppl 2):150-6.

Kanehisa H, Ikegawa S, Fukunaga T (1994) Comparison of muscle cross-sectional area and strength between untrained women and men. *European Journal of Applied Physiology: Occupational Physiology* 68(2): 148-54.

Kendall F P, McCreary E K, Provance P G (1993) *Muscles Testing and Function*. 4th Edition. Lippincott Williams & Wilkins, Philadelphia PA.

Kraemer W J, Ratamess N A (2005) Hormonal Responses and Adaptations to Resistance Exercise and Training. *Journal of Sports Medicine* 35(4):339-61.

Layne JE, Nelson ME (1999) The effects of progressive resistance training on bone density: a review. *Medicine and Science in Sports and Exercise* 31(1):25-30.

Laughton et al (2003) Ageing, muscle activity and balance control: physiologic changes associated with balance impairment. *Journal of Gait and Posture* 18:101-108.

Leetun D T, Ireland M L, Willson J D, Ballantyne B T, Davis I M (2004) Core stability measures as risk factors for lower extremity injuries in athletes. *Medicine and Science in Sports and Exercise* 36(6):926-934.

Lindle R S et al (1997) Age and gender comparisons of muscle strength in 654 women and men aged 20-93. *Journal of Applied Physiology* 83: 1581-1587.

Lipski E (2000) *Digestive Wellness*. Keats, Los Angeles.

Martinson EW (1990) Benefits of exercise for the treatment of depression. *Journal of Sports Medicine* 9(6):380-9.

McArdle W D, Katch F, Katch V L (2001) *Exercise Physiology: Energy, Nutrition and Human Performance*, 5th Edition. Lippincott Williams and Wilkins, Baltimore MA.

McCann IL, Holmes DS (1984) Influence of aerobic exercise on depression. *Journal of Personal Social Psychology* 46(5):1142-7.

McCartney N (1998) Role of resistance training in heart disease. *Medicine and Science in Sports and Exercise* 30(10):S396-S402 .

McGill S (2006) *Ultimate Back Fitness and Performance*. 3rd Edition, Wabuno Publishers, Ontario, Canada.

Miller A E, Macdougall J D, Tarnopolsky M A, Sale D G (1993) Gender differences in strength and muscle fiber characteristics. *European Journal of Applied Physiology: Occupational Physiology* 66(3): 254-62.

Myer G D, Ford K R, Palumbo J P, Hewett T E (2005) Neuromuscular training improves performance and lower-extremity biomechanics in female athletes. *Journal of Strength and Conditioning Research* 19(1):51-60.

Oka RK et al (2000) Impact of a home-based walking and resistance training programme on quality of life in patients with heart failure. *American Journal of Cardiology* 85(3):365-9.

Petruzello SJ, Landers DM, Hatfield BD, Kubitz KA, Salazar W (1991) A meta-analysis on the anxiety reducing effects of acute and chronic exercise. Outcomes and mechanisms. *Journal of Sports Medicine* 11(3):143-82.

Pitt-Brooke J – Ed. (1998) Rehabilitation of Movement: Theoretical Basis of Clinical Practice, WB Saunders, London.

Poirer P, Despres J P (2001) Exercise in weight management of Obesity. *Journal of Clinical Cardiology* 19(3):459-70.

Poliquin C (1989) Theory and Methodology of Strength Training (Part 1) Sports Coach.

Porterfield J A, Derosa C (1998) *Mechanical Low Back Pain: Perspectives in Functional Anatomy.* Philadelphia PA: W B Saunders.

Pu et al (2001) Randomised trial of progressive resistance training to counteract the myopathy of chronic heart failure. *Journal of Applied Physiology* 90:2341-2350.

Raglin JS, Morgan WP (1987) Influence of exercise and quiet rest on state anxiety and blood pressure. *Medicine and Science in Sports and Exercise* 19(5):456-63.

Reinking M F, Alexander L E (2005) Prevalence of disordered-eating behaviours in undergraduate female collegiate athletes and non-athletes. *Journal of Athletic Training* 40(1): 47-51.

Richardson C A, Jull G, Hodges P, Hide J (1999) *Therapeutic Exercise for Spinal Stabilisation and Low Back Pain: Scientific basis and clinical approach.* Churchill Livingstone, Edinburgh.

Sahrmann S (2002) *Diagnosis and Treatment of Movement Impairment Syndromes.* St Louis MI: Mosby.

Schmidt R A, Wrisberg C A (2000) *Motor Learning and Performance.* 2nd Edition. Human Kinetics, Champaign IL.

Segar ML et al (1998) The effect of aerobic exercise on self-esteem and depressive and anxiety symptoms among breast cancer survivors. *Oncology and Nursing Forum* 25(4):654.

Siff M C (2003) *Supertraining*, Supertraining Institute, Denver USA.

Soukup JT, Kovaleski JE (1993) A review of the effects of resistance training for individuals with diabetes mellitus. *Journal of Diabetes Education* 19(4):307-12.

Spring H, Illi U, Kunz H, Rothlin K, Schneider W, Tritschler T (1991) *Stretching and Strengthening Exercises*. Thieme Medical Publishers Inc, New York NY.

Sysko R, Walsh B T, Schebendach J, Wilson G T (2005) Eating behaviour among women with Anorexia Nervosa. *American Journal of Clinical Nutrition* 82(2): 296-301.

Talbot S (2002) *The Cortisol Connection – Why stress makes you fat and what you can do about it.* Hunter House, Alameda CA.

Tippet S R, Voight M R (1995) *Functional Progressions for Sports Rehabilitation*, Human Kinetics, Champaign IL.

Willoughby DS (2001) *ACSM Position Stand – Resistance training and the older adult.* American College of Sports Medicine – Current Comments.

Zatsiorsky V M (1995) Science and Practice of Strength Training, Human Kinetics, Champaign, IL. USA.

www.heartstats.org/atozpage.asp?id=1912 – Age-standardised prevalence of diagnosed diabetes by sex and household income, 2003, England (Table)
Source: Health Survey for England 2003 (2004).

www.bhf.org.uk - British Heart Foundation website.

www.diabetes.org.uk - Diabetes U.K website.

www.mercola.com - Dr Joseph Mercola holistic health website and newsletter.

www.nlm.nih.gov - National Library of Medicine.

GLOSSARY AND ABBREVIATIONS

abdominals	See *rectus abdominis*, *obliques* and *transversus abdominis*.
aerobic	Literally, 'with oxygen'. Aerobic exercise involves working muscles supplied with sufficient oxygen.
anaerobic	Literally, 'without oxygen'. Anaerobic exercise involves using muscles before the heart can circulate more oxygen to help them work.
antioxidants	Molecules present in certain foods that counteract the effects of some oxidant *free radicals* in the body.
calcium	Naturally occurring alkaline metal in the body, used chiefly for growth, maintenance and strength of bones and teeth. Lack of calcium can contribute to *osteoporosis*.
free radicals	Molecules present in certain substances that can have a damaging effect on cells in the body.
hip flexors	The muscles we use to keep our pelvis in position and for movement of the hips and legs. The iliacus and psoas major (known jointly as the iliopsoas) are at the front of the hip; the psoas major runs from the lower spine, through the pelvis, to the top of the leg.
hypertrophy	(hypertrophy) Gaining muscle through exercise.
insulin	Hormone produced in the pancreas that attaches to cells, regulating the absorption of carbohydrates; dictates blood sugar levels and fat storage in the body.
interval training	A period of hard physical activity followed by a period of less intensive exercise called 'active recovery'.
ischemia	A lack of oxygen in the body, usually as a result of *tachycardia*.
magnesium	Metallic element available in supplements to combat insomnia, muscle cramps, stress and fatigue.
obliques (external/internal)	Abdominal muscles that crisscross the mid-section providing stability, lateral movement and rotation.
Omega 3/Omega 6	Fatty acids used by the body for new cell production, and which produce enzymes to maintain joint and organ function.
osteoporosis	Decrease in bone density leading to fragility, through cellular damage and/or a lack of *calcium*.
pelvic floor	The muscles at the base of the pelvis, intersected by the urethra, rectum and (in females) vagina. Controls urinary and sexual functions.
PNF	Proprioceptive Neuromuscular Facilitation: PNF stretches are designed to get the most out of a muscle by honing function of *proprioceptors*.
proprioceptors	Tiny nervous sensors in joints and muscles that relay information back to the brain about joint position and muscle extension to regulate posture, movement and balance.
radial pulse	The pulse located in the back of the wrist in line with the base of the thumb.
rectus abdominis	The 'six-pack' muscle which stretches from the ribs at the front of the torso to the pelvis.
RPE	Rate of Perceived Exertion: a self-regulated scale from one to 10 to gauge whether you are doing light, moderate or hard exercise.
serotonin	Hormone released by the brain to initiate sleep. Also thought to affect anger, body temperature, mood, sexuality, and appetite.
tachycardia	An abnormally high resting heart rate.
transversus abdominis (TVA)	The deepest of the abdominal muscles, running round the torso like a corset. Used predominantly in function for expiration.
tryptophan	Amino acid in certain foods that triggers release of *serotonin*.
tyramine	Amino acid compound that releases stimulants into the body – present in caffeine, chocolate and tobacco et al.

INDEX